IMPROVING

HEALTHCARE WITH

BETTER BUILDING

DESIGN

IMPROVING HEALTHCARE WITH BETTER BUILDING DESIGN

Sara O. Marberry, Editor

ACHE Management Series

Health Administration Press

Your board, staff, or clients may also benefit from this book's insight. For more information on quantity discounts, contact the Health Administration Press Marketing Manager at (312) 424-9470.

10   09   08   07   06   5   4   3   2   1

Library of Congress Cataloging-in-Publication Data

Improving healthcare with better buidling design / Sara O. marberry, editor.
    p. cm.
  Includes bibliographical references and index.
  ISBN-10: 1-56793-249-5
  ISBN-13: 978-1-56793-249-2
  1. Hospitals—Design and construction.   I. Marberry, Sara O., 1959–
RA967.I53 2005
362.11—dc22

                                           2005052520

The paper used in this publication meets the minimum requirements of American National Standard for Information Sciences—Permanence of Paper for Printed Library Materials, ANSI Z39.48-1984. ∞™

Acquisitions manager: Janet Davis; project manager: Melissa A. Rompesky; cover design: Gregory Kerkman

Health Administration Press
A division of the Foundation
    of the American College of
    Healthcare Executives
One North Franklin Street
Suite 1700
Chicago, IL 60606-3346
(312) 424-2800

Cover photograph used with permission.
Parrish Medical Center, Titusville, FL
Photography: Scott McDonald/Hedrich Blessing
Architecture: Earl Swensson Associates

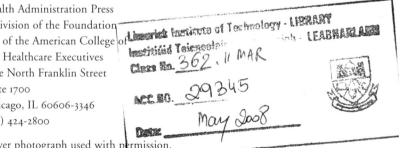

DEDICATION

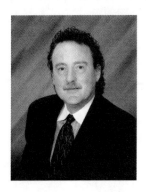

Russell C. Coile, Jr.

This book is dedicated to Russell C. Coile, Jr., who passed away November 10, 2003, at age 60. A long-time member of The Center for Health Design's board of directors, Russ was a dear colleague who was instrumental in shaping and guiding our mission for more than a decade. He was the one who came up with the idea for this book, and he helped to develop it up until a month before his death.

His wit, humor, and intellect are sorely missed by all those who knew him. As one of the country's leading healthcare forecasters, Russ was rarely wrong in his predictions. His annual top-ten predictions for the healthcare field were 90 percent accurate. A prolific author and sought-after speaker, he had a way with words—for example, describing healthcare's new consumers as "Boomers, BoBos, HealthSeekers, and the Wired Retired."

Russ was a champion of the built environment's impact on the quality of healthcare. He often wrote about it in his best-selling books, newsletter, and the award-winning *Futurescan* reports he authored for the American Hospital Association and American College of Healthcare Executives. A celebrated speaker, he also helped enlighten many at conferences and meetings across the United States.

It is our hope that this book will help fulfill the dream that Russ shared with us—to transform healthcare settings into healing environments that contribute to health and improve outcomes through the creative use of evidence-based design.

Contents

Acknowledgments   ix

List of Figures and Tables   xi

1   The Opportunity Is Now   1
Rosalyn Cama, FASID

2   What Patients Want: Designing and Delivering
Health Services that Respect Personhood   15
Paul Alexander Clark, M.P.A., and
Mary P. Malone, M.S., J.D.

3   The Environment's Impact on Stress   37
Roger S. Ulrich, Ph.D.; Craig Zimring, Ph.D.;
Xiaobo Quan, and Anjali Joseph

4   The Environment's Impact on Safety   63
Craig Zimring, Ph.D.; Roger S. Ulrich, Ph.D.;
Anjali Joseph, and Xiaobo Quan

5   Environmentally Responsible Hospitals   81
Greg Roberts, AIA, FCSI, ACHA, LEED AP,
and Robin Guenther, AIA, LEED AP

6   Designing a Better Environment   109
Jain Malkin

7   The Compelling Business Case for Better
Buildings   125
Blair Sadler, J.D., D. Kirk Hamilton, FAIA, FACHA;
Derek Parker, FAIA, RIBA, FACHA; and
Leonard L. Berry, Ph.D.

8   Cultural Transformation and Design   145
D. Kirk Hamilton, FAIA, FACHA, and
Robin Diane Orr, M.P.H.

9   The Vision Starts at the Top   161
     Sara O. Marberry

     About the Contributors   177

     About the Center for Health Design   185

     Index   187

Acknowledgments

WRITING OF THIS book was made possible with assistance from Turner Healthcare. Special thanks to Robert Levine at Turner for his support and encouragement of The Center for Health Design's work; without his help, this book might have never been written.

A big thanks to all the contributing authors, who believe so strongly in The Center's work that they donated their time and expertise to create this one-of-a-kind book.

Particular thanks also to the following individuals: Debra J. Levin, president, The Center for Health Design, for being such a terrific colleague and friend; Janet R. Davis, acquisitions editor, Health Administration Press, for making the publishing process so enjoyable; Leonard R. Berry, Ph.D., contributing author and professor at Texas A&M University, for providing thoughtful, invaluable editorial guidance; Richard J. Marberry, my husband, for keeping the home fires burning while I toiled away in my office; and Phares and Harriet O'Daffer, my parents, for always being there and giving me the genes to be a writer.

List of Figures and Tables

Chapter 1
Table 1.1:   Matrix for Uniform Data Collection   10

Chapter 2
Figure 2.1:   Maslow's Hierarchy of Needs   17
Table 2.1:   Strongest Correlations to Patients' Loyalty   20
Table 2.2:   Patients' Greatest Priorities for Health Services   22
Figure 2.2:   Patient Loyalty and Satisfaction   26
Table 2.3:   Analysis of Patient Satisfaction Response
              Category Percentage by Percentile Rank for
              Inpatient Acute Care, 2004   27
Figure 2.3:   Average Percentage "Very Good" Ratings, by
              Overall Percentile Rank   27

Chapter 3
[none]

Chapter 4
[none]

Chapter 5

Figure 5.1:   Interrelationship Between Environmental
              Pollution and Healthcare   83
Figure 5.2:   The Triple Bottom Line for Health   85
Figure 5.3:   Applying the Triple Bottom Line Approach
              at the Community Level   91
Figure 5.4:   The Integral Framework of Socially
              Responsible Organizations   99
Figure 5.5:   The Integral Framework Applied to
              Healthcare Decision Makers   101

Chapter 6
[none]

Chapter 7

Table 7.1:   Incremental Cost to Achieve a
              Better Building   130
Table 7.2:   Financial Impact of Design Decisions   133

Chapter 8

Figure 8.1:   Broad Cultural Roles Healthcare Organizations
              Might Adopt   148
Figure 8.2:   Cultural Transformation Checklist   156

Chapter 9
[none]

CHAPTER 1

The Opportunity Is Now

Rosalyn Cama, FASID

THIS BOOK IS intended to change the way healthcare leaders look at building design for healthcare and the effect its design has on human behavior. In most corporate segments the understanding of this phenomenon is clear. In healthcare, however, the case to date has been relatively weak. It is our intention to address hospital buildings, their design features, and resulting behavioral changes that affect outcomes relative to health and healing, organizational efficiencies, and improved financial performance.

CURRENT ENVIRONMENT FOR CHANGE

The current healthcare environment offers many opportunities for positive change. Cost of care and expectations of delivery are misaligned, operational inefficiencies abound, and the fussiest of generations (baby boomers) has exploded onto the scene as primary customers. In addition, life expectancy continues to increase, the ability to feel young and stay active is expected as age-related illnesses intensify, and new technology is driving an unyielding magnitude of operational and procedural changes. What's more, labor shortages grow in many clinical areas as job demands move healthcare workers' tasks away from the very act of giving care, safety protocols and quality-of-care issues remain unstandardized, outmoded facilities lack an infrastructure to accommodate new technologies, and many organizations struggle with the issue of whether to remodel or replace.

The environment is ripe for change, so how will these changes occur, and what motivating factor will initiate them in a responsible way? New building projects often drive some of these discussions, but little research has been done to see exactly how coupling cultural changes with a new facility can drive massive behavioral changes, particularly in light of the above burning issues.

Healthcare construction spending in the United States is estimated to be $16.7 billion in 2005, rising to about $18.8 billion in 2009 (McGraw Hill Construction 2005) and to $33 billion by 2010 (Babwin 2002). Nearly three-fourths of chief financial officers surveyed by the Healthcare Financial Management Association (2004) said that they will increase their hospital's capital spending over the next five years. In addition, the pressures of an aging population, increasing life expectancy, rising fertility rates, and continuing immigration could result in a nationwide shortage of 150,000 to 200,000 beds by 2012 (Carpenter 2003). A wide-open opportunity to introduce change therefore exists. But should change be initiated strictly for the sake of change? Absolutely not.

ADVOCATES FOR AN INFORMED PROCESS FOR CHANGE

The Center for Health Design (The Center), a nonprofit research and advocacy organization, has taken on the task of initiating the needed changes in healthcare design. Founded in 1993 by a group of healthcare and design professionals, The Center's mission is to transform healthcare settings into healing environments that improve outcomes through the creative use of evidence-based design. A healing environment is one that is based on research or evidence used to inform design decisions. The research comes from the fields of evolutionary biology, neurosciences, psychoneuroimmunology (the effect of the emotions on the immune system and environmental psychology). The common theme is the reduction of stress. The

Center also has a vision for a future in which healing environments are recognized as a vital part of therapeutic treatment and in which the design of healthcare settings contributes to health rather than adds to the burden of stress.

In establishing its mission and vision The Center knew it would have to create a win-win situation for healthcare executives and board members. To that end, its efforts have to be aligned with the strategic initiatives of healthcare organizations. Therefore, it is important to identify just what those initiatives are.

The Center's board articulates these initiatives in its value proposition, which is based on the fact that building or renovating a healthcare facility is a major capital investment. For this reason The Center believes that the leading healthcare organizations of the twenty-first century will be those that are passionately committed to providing optimal environments for their patients, staff, and visitors. Such organizations will realize sustained strategic business advantages over their competitors by

- improving the quality of care for their patients;
- enhancing their operational efficiency and productivity;
- increasing their market share by attracting more patients;
- being better able to recruit and retain highly qualified staff; and
- increasing philanthropic, corporate, and community support.

The realization of these advantages is The Center's wish for every healthcare organization, particularly for every healthcare organization that undertakes a new building project.

WHERE IT ALL STARTED

Although The Center's focus has always been clear, the healthcare industry has not always been ready to undertake the change it advocates. Early on The Center reached out to an audience of approximately 25,000 healthcare and design professionals who used its formula for building a healing environment. That formula was based on a simple breakdown of available research at the time. Roger Ulrich, Ph.D., an environmental researcher at Texas A&M University (see Chapters 3 and 4), categorized all research available at the time into five areas:

1. Access to nature
2. Control
3. Positive distractions
4. Social support
5. Environmental stressers

This formula was the basis for the construction of many fine healthcare facilities that have served as examples of best practices for many years.

Early Research

During this time The Center sought out researchers in the fields of environmental psychology, neuroscience, evolutionary biology, and psychoneuroimmunology. These were the academicians who were researching the very outcomes that showed a correlation between the environment and human behavior. Audiences at healthcare design conferences in the 1990s were left to establish their own methodology for applying these nuggets of valuable knowledge. Without doubt, a generation of healthcare designers, while doing little or no research themselves, developed a pattern of design vocabulary steeped in this rich academic knowledge.

In 1997 The Center published a report compiling all such available knowledge (Rubin, Owens, and Golden 1997). Although extensive and led by a respected Johns Hopkins research team, the report revealed only 84 significant research studies. This landmark study sent The Center on a journey to build a research agenda that would fill in the many knowledge gaps.

The Center next partnered with the Picker Institute to conduct a focus-group-driven study to determine what mattered most to consumers of healthcare services in acute, ambulatory, and long-term care areas of service. This report found a commonality in all areas of healthcare service (McRae 1998) and distilled consumers' preferences for the facilities in which they would receive care as those that would

- facilitate a connection to staff;
- be conducive to well-being;
- be convenient and accessible;
- be confidential and private;
- be caring for their families;
- be considerate of their impairments; and
- be close to nature

Chapter 2 expands on this knowledge and translates it to health services by exploring the idea of personhood and asking what is it that people want, need, and love.

Evidence-based Healthcare Design

Armed with the Picker research, The Center launched a broader agenda into the realm of evidence-based design. Wanting to discover how best to equip those responsible for building healthcare institutions, The Center took a close look at the Institute of Medicine (IOM.) report on improving the quality of care delivery. The IOM report identified six factors for best practices. The Center looked carefully at these factors and determined which design features would contribute to the changes in behavior needed to achieve the necessary shift in care delivery (The Center 2002):

1. **Patient centered:** If the focus is on the patient, the building design must reflect and support this by honoring the individual and respecting choice. Patient-centered design features include private rooms, positive distractions, accommodation for family members, and ways to access information.

2. **Timely:** The building environment can contribute to the timeliness of care by facilitating access to patients and communication. Related design features include the layout of units, nurse station design, conference areas, and resource areas.
3. **Efficient:** The building design can reduce waste in the healthcare system by facilitating reduced transfers and increased work efficiency. Efficiency design features include decentralized nursing and universal patient rooms.
4. **Equitable:** The building design can contribute to equitable care by being family centered and accessible to all. Design features that address equity include single patient rooms with accommodations for family members, respite areas, site location and layout, and welcoming, private admitting areas.
5. **Effective:** The building design can help the delivery of care to be more effective through improved sleep quality, decreased infections, lower stress, and increased staff satisfaction. Design features that address care effectiveness include private patient rooms; location of hand-washing facilities; elimination of environmental stressers such as noise, glare, odor, and poor indoor air quality; better wayfinding; supportive staff work areas; staff lounges; and positive distractions.
6. **Safe:** The building design can help the delivery of care to be more safe by facilitating reduced patient falls, medical errors, and infections. Design features that address safety include decentralized nursing stations, room layout, elimination of environmental stressers, location of hand-washing facilities, materials selection, and improved air quality.

These examples, delivered in an ongoing executive lecture series sponsored by Turner Healthcare, have been shared with healthcare executives and senior-level design professionals across the United States. At a minimum these examples constitute the informed base of knowledge a design team needs to give its building project to allow clinicians to provide quality care. These lectures have spurred great interest in the area of evidence-based design, and many field-study projects, known as Pebble Projects (see discussion in t he next section), have grown from these discussions.

MORE DATA IN SOME AREAS THAN OTHERS

In 2004, with funding from The Robert Wood Johnson Foundation, The Center commissioned a new search of available research in this area (Ulrich and Zimring 2004). Remarkably, 600 studies were revealed, a significant increase over the 84 discovered in the Johns Hopkins search just six years earlier. The specifics of this research work are noted in chapters 3 and 4.

Particularly useful to both healthcare executives and design professionals is Ulrich and Zimring's categorization of the studies into four subsets:

1. Reduction of staff stress and fatigue
2. Improvement in patient safety
3. Reduction of patient stress
4. Improvement of overall healthcare quality

Even more useful as a tool are the four scorecards they created for each of these subsets, ranking topics according to a five-star rating system (Ulrich 2004). These scorecards identify five-star areas, such as the need for private rooms, as so compelling that design or project teams and healthcare executives no longer need to debate the issue. However, in areas in which little research has been conducted—those related to staff efficiencies, for example—a minimally starred category gives The Center a cue that research is needed to prove or disprove design solutions. If these data have already been collected, it is easier to justify decisions to board members, senior management, and even members of the community, especially if more money than originally anticipated must be spent on a hospital project. Chapter 7 uses some of these data to make the business case for constructing a better building.

AN INFORMED APPROACH TO DESIGN

So what is evidence-based design? Evidence-based design is a deliberate attempt to base design decisions on quantitative and sometimes qualitative research. When we look at the specific outcomes a healthcare organization can expect as the result of design recommendations, the literature suggests the following parameters:

- Patient-related outcomes
- Staff satisfaction
- Quality
- Safety
- Operational efficiency
- Financial performance

This knowledge arms senior healthcare managers and design teams with practical applications for design solutions and, in a relatively conservative way, mitigates any risks associated with known design solutions. These parameters allow a clear understanding of behaviors that cause certain outcomes and design solutions that support those behaviors. The innovative healthcare organization has a sturdy platform from which to hypothesize and determine the next best way to solve for better outcomes.

Competitive Advantage

The Center's Pebble Project has become one of the world's largest field-study projects in the area of healthcare design. Started in 2000, the initiative was created and so named to create a ripple effect at the planning tables of all hospitals undergoing a renovation or a new building project. The literature and conference discussions alone would not be enough to stir the minds of these hospital CEOs, board members, facility directors, and other senior-level business decision makers. However, if a group of peers measured and shared their specific outcomes, maybe this audience would join The Center's dialog.

To get started, a prototype project at San Diego Children's Hospital was used to establish a research model. Under the expertise of James Varni, Ph.D., a matrix was created to allow for a uniform collection of data (see Table 1.1). This matrix also allows The Center to see where trends are occurring in behavioral shifts; with honest reporting, methodologies established also identify where design features are not performing as well. The matrix allows for flexibility in studying groups or subsets thereof. It also allows for flexibility in outcomes.

At first the desired outcomes fell into three categories related to clinical or health considerations, organizational, and then financial areas. Many of the early Pebbles were interested in satisfaction and quality issues, safety, and error omission rates; with this level of consciousness about the impact the environment has on humankind, they have become interested in the effects on our natural environment as well. The time has come for healthcare organizations to be good corporate citizens and use sustainable, green-building practices to create healthier facilities that do not harm the natural environment or people. Chapter 5 discusses in detail the impact of the built environment on the health of its occupants, local communities, and global ecosystems.

More than 30 healthcare organizations have participated in the Pebble Project research initiative since 2000. (A list of current participants can be found on The Center's web site at www.healthdesign.org.) Projects vary in size and type and are in various stages; participants include entire acute care hospitals, specific patient units, clinics, and long-term care facilities.

To date, five hospitals have reported on research findings, and more are collecting data as they finish their projects. The beauty of this field-study project is the continuum of evidence that is mounting, with attention to the top issues in the current care-delivery climate. As the premise for the engagement of these providers is to follow a specific research methodology, the findings will be clean. The hospitals are allowed to develop their own research agendas with their design teams with the facilitation of a Center researcher. Representatives from each participating organization attend two

Table 1.1: Matrix for Uniform Data Collection

Outcome Researched	Comparative Group				
	Patients (S, G, or A)	Employees/ Physicians (S, G, or A)	Family/ Visitors (S, G, or A)	Community	Organization/ Institution
Clinical/technical outcomes		N/A	N/A	N/A	N/A
Economic/ financial resource utilization					N/A
Operational improvements				N/A	
Satisfaction, quality of life, cultural assessment					
Safety/error reduction outcomes			N/A		
Environmental/ sustainability					
Other measurable outcomes					

S = Same (identical) group of patients, families, or employees pre- and post-intervention.
G = Group (type/group) of patients, families, or employees pre- and post-intervention.
A = All (the entire population) of patients, families, or employees pre- and post-intervention.

yearly colloquials and one annual conference to share research-based ideas that are applicable to their design hypotheses.

After they analyze their goals, develop hypotheses, search the literature, translate those findings into new and innovative solutions, and then measure results on occupancy, participants too must share their findings with the healthcare industry at large through publication in a peer-reviewed journal. What this does for the early adopters, who are not interested in innovating, is provide a current base of knowledge that will mitigate the risk associated with expensive unsubstantiated trends. Right now we can only look to best practices that have come to the fore in the last five years, which means they were designed with thinking that is at least ten years old. The Pebble Project allows for a steady flow of thinking supported by rigorous findings that will spur advancement in an industry that has been slow to progress.

Armed with these data, The Center's Environmental Standards Council (ESC) takes this knowledge to a more regulatory level. Working with the Joint Commission on Accreditation of Healthcare Organizations (JCAHO), ESC has created evidence-based examples for JCAHO's Environment of Care chapter. The volunteer healthcare and design professionals who serve on this council have also worked diligently with the American Institute of Architects in the revision of the "Guidelines for Design and Construction of Hospital and Health Care Facilities." This group is now establishing relationships with medical manufacturers to share the data as they pertain to product development and the role products play in healing at all levels.

IT TAKES LEADERSHIP

Without doubt, strong leadership drives all Pebble Projects. Defining that leadership is not the goal of The Center, but it is a criterion for admission into this elite group of evidence-based projects. (Chapter 9 tells the story of three CEOs whose strong leadership and vision helped create extraordinary projects.)

Being a strong leader means leading with a core set of values. According to Leonard Berry, Ph.D. (1999), at Texas A&M University (see Chapter 7), the "more these values tap into employees' own core values, the more they guide individual decision making and inspire personal achievement." Having core values energizes an organization and gets people behind a cause. Berry acknowledges that leaders perform other important roles, but they lead with values by

- Articulating the dream
- Defining organizational success
- Cultivating leadership in others
- Asserting values in tough times
- Challenging the status quo
- Encouraging the heart

Berry also identifies nine drivers of sustainable success in service businesses. At the center is values-driven leadership, which gives root to the other eight drivers:

1. Strategic focus
2. Executional excellence
3. Control of destiny
4. Trust-based relationships
5. Investment in employee success
6. Acting small
7. Brand cultivation
8. Generosity

It should also be noted that many building projects require a cultural transformation. To use an analogy from the theater, if the stage changes, so must the show. And in many cases cultural transformation occurs as the building is being designed or even after it is built. Yet, as Chapter 8 explains, it is better to design the organization before you design the building. The performance outcomes and financial risks are simply too important to ignore this advice.

When history is recorded, missed opportunities become clear. Will these issues be resolved in a clear and succinct way? We are at a point at which changes to our healthcare system need to occur. Courage and a lot of reassurance are needed to innovate in an industry that has so much at risk. The Center's goal is to arm healthcare leaders with risk-averse tools in the form of evidence-based knowledge to take advantage of current opportunities.

REFERENCES

Babwin, D. 2002. "Building Boom." *Hospitals & Health Networks* March: 48–54.

Berry, L. 1999. *Discovering the Soul of Service.* New York: Free Press.

Carpenter, D. 2003. "Behind the Boom." *Health Facilities Management.* [Online information.] www.hfmmagazine.com.

The Center for Health Design. 2002. "Competing by Design." Executive program sponsored by Turner Healthcare, Indianapolis, IN, October 11.

Healthcare Financial Management Association. 2004. "Financing the Future. Report Three." Westchester, IL: HFMA.

Institute of Medicine. 2001. *Crossing the Quality Chasm: A New Health System for the 21st Century.* Washington, DC: IOM.

McGraw Hill Construction. 2005. *Dodge Market Analysis Value Report 2005 Q1.* New York: McGraw Hill.

McRae, S. 1998. *Consumer Perceptions of the Healthcare Environment: An Investigation to Determine What Matters.* Concord, CA: The Center for Health Design.

Rubin, H. R., A. J. Owens, and G. Golden, 1997. "An Investigation to Determine Whether the Built Environment Affects Patients' Medical Outcomes." Concord, CA. The Center for Health Design.

Ulrich, R. 2004. "Effects of Healthcare Architecture on Medical Outcomes." Presented at Designing the 21st Century Hospital, Leadership Discussion Sponsored by The Center for Health Design and the Robert Wood Johnson Foundation, Washington, DC June 3.

Ulrich, R., and C. Zimring. 2004. *The Role of the Physical Environment in the Hospital of the 21st Century.* Concord, CA: The Center for Health Design.

What Patients Want: Designing and Delivering Health Services that Respect Personhood

Paul Alexander Clark, M.P.A.
Mary P. Malone, M.S., J.D.

A PERSON IS an embodied, intelligent being with the free will to act in fulfillment of his human needs (Ashley and O'Rourke 2002). A person is dynamic, changing, and inextricably linked to the human needs that possess all of us. The way in which we fulfill our human needs makes us who we are as people and constitutes our personhood.

As healthcare providers, you are not serving patients; you are serving people. You are designing and delivering services to meet the needs of normal people at the most difficult times in their lives. You are serving sick, lonely, suffering, scared, distressed, and worried people whose planned life journeys were irrevocably altered.

We often are asked, "What do patients or patients' families think?" as if patients and their relatives were somehow a different species with different thoughts or feelings than normal humans. We are asked this question because the traditional notion of a patient is someone to whom we do things; someone who needs to be fixed; someone expected to give up at least a portion of her free will to undergo the clinician's decided course of treatment; someone treated, manipulated, and in short dominated—at least in the traditional, perhaps unconscious, view.

In planning, designing, and delivering health services we often make the mistake of moving directly to patient, or even customer, concepts instead of considering human beings in the context of their natural existence. Those who have designed and innovated the world's greatest products and services did not conceptualize an abstract customer, but rather were completely attuned to the reality of life and fundamental human needs.

Now that we have begun to align our thought with the concept of personhood, the questions healthcare leaders and managers should ask in designing and delivering a health service include

- What is it that people need?
- What is it that people want?
- What is it that people love?

MASLOW'S HIERARCHY: SAFETY AT ALL COSTS

Perhaps no one is more greatly associated with human needs than Abraham Maslow. Maslow (1987) grouped all human needs into a hierarchy: (1) physiological, (2) safety, (3) social, (4) esteem, and (5) self-actualization (see Figure 2.1). At each level a person must satisfy needs before striving to fulfill needs at the next level. A person must fulfill physiological needs before pursuing safety, social, esteem, and self-actualization needs. Physiological needs include food; water; clean air; and basic health services, such as life-saving interventions. Next, a person needs to feel and be safe through a secure environment, protection from harm, trust in those who surround him, and comfort or peace of mind in the knowledge that these needs will be fulfilled in the future. Social needs come next as we search for interaction, attention, and relationships, often categorized as psychosocial needs. Esteem represents what we derive from our actions and relationships: understanding, love, and emotional and spiritual support. Finally, self-actualization occurs when we operate at a fully charged, high level and experience the feeling of fulfilled purpose and meaning.

Maslow's popular hierarchy matches well with how health services have been designed and delivered in the past 50 years. The fore-

Figure 2.1: Maslow's Hierarchy of Needs

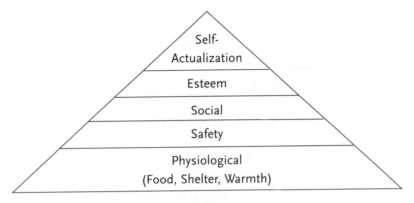

Source: Maslow, Abraham, MOTIVATION AND PERSONALITY, 1987. Reprinted by permission of Pearson Education Inc., Upper Saddle River, New Jersey.

most priority among healthcare professionals is to first, do no harm. Indeed, as laypersons undoubtedly agree, we do no want to be sick, and we definitely do not want to get sicker. We want to at least maintain our current bodily integrity; we do not want to be harmed. The Institute of Medicine's ([IOM] 2001) definition of quality reflects Maslow's hierarchy, declaring that healthcare must be

1. safe,
2. effective,
3. timely,
4. efficient,
5. equitable, and
6. patient centered.

Although IOM's finding that between 44,000 and 98,000 patients die annually in the United States as a result of preventable medical errors has heightened healthcare industry professionals' attention to safety and security, we have yet to see evidence that this has changed the perceptions of patients or the public. The consensus explanation is that patients and family members consider adequate technical quality to be a given. Only in the absence of technical quality do we notice and prioritize it. Many studies indicate that patients and families desire a certain threshold of safety, security, and technical quality; once this minimum standard has been reached, other factors or needs become paramount.

Maslow would lead us to believe that traditional amenities and technical aspects of quality should be of the greatest importance to patients. This notion is not supported by the data (as we will see later), nor does it reflect the experiences of real life in dire and difficult circumstances. Powerful human emotions, such as love, humor, and spirituality, emerge forcefully when life becomes endangered. Many irrational decisions are made based on emotional needs (Hastie and Dawes 2001). Mathematician Blaise Pascal (1623–1662) observed, "The heart has its reasons which reason knows nothing of" (Pascal 1941). Humans today continue to risk security for love. We need humor when faced with difficulty. We seek to touch the divine when our lives look most bleak.

The reasons for this disconnect between the priorities suggested by Maslow's theory and healthcare consumers' actual behavior may lie in the fact that Maslow intended his hierarchy to explain human motivation. His findings were based on a series of case studies observing high-performing individuals. It is important to understand the context of the theory: these were psychological studies intended to answer the question of what motivates humans to achieve high levels of performance. As Maslow's hierarchy is a theory of motivation based on high-achieving, healthy individuals, it may be that the prioritization of human needs shifts and changes like a kaleidoscope when humans undergo difficult or life-threatening experiences.[1]

Although it possesses undeniable intuitive appeal, Maslow's hierarchy is inadequate in fulfilling patients' wants and needs. Nevertheless, the practice of healthcare management has strictly adhered to Maslow's hierarchy. Senior management often only concentrates entirely on safety, with patients' wants and needs only an afterthought. The result? Limited vision and lack of openness to innovation. In a recent conversation a healthcare CEO stated bluntly,

"I don't care if patients have a window; I want them to be safe."
Why can't patients have both?

VOICE OF THE PATIENT: TOTAL HEALTHCARE SERVICES DESIGN

We drew from the largest single-method database of patients' assessments of their healthcare experiences. The data include the responses of more than nine million patients in 2004. Patients' perspectives on acute inpatient care, outpatient care, emergency departments, physician offices, home health care, and nursing homes were included using the approach of scientific reductionism—that is, reducing what people find most important in healthcare to its most elemental parts. In other words, across different healthcare service settings, medical specialties, organizational characteristics, and patient characteristics, what commonalities emerge that tell us people consider certain universal needs most important when receiving any health service? The answer to this question will isolate factors critical to patient loyalty and improving satisfaction. With these results, healthcare managers can take the next step in designing health services to truly foster personhood.

Table 2.1 lists the top five patient assessments with the strongest correlations to patient loyalty for acute inpatient care, outpatient care, emergency department, medical practice, and nursing home settings. The themes of staff response, demonstration of care and concern, clinicians' communication (information, explanation), and attention or sensitivity to special or personal needs are strong. Almost everything important to patients' loyalty occurs within the therapeutic encounter. What happens when patient and clinician meet is of paramount importance to whether the patient will recommend or return to that organization, facility, or provider.

Many of these assessments are worded slightly differently for the particular patient populations, but behind them are universal human needs. For example, "special or personal needs," "staff cared about you as a person," and "our sensitivity to your needs" all point to a desire that clinicians personalize the encounter and attend to what makes us unique individuals.

It is also important to note the difference between actual physical comfort and staff concern for comfort or other assessments of physical needs. These key words indicate that people care more that providers demonstrate concern or caring behaviors than the actual physical sensations they experience. People do not blame the clinician or organization for being sick, even if, as in the case of medical errors, the illness is the organization's fault. People do blame others for not showing that they care.

Another important distinction is the provision of information. This gets to the how and what. What information are patients receiving? Do they understand this information? Do they want this information? Is this really what they want to know about, or is this what the institution wants to tell them? What does the patient want to know? An organization that respects personhood in providing information would ask the person what information they want to know instead of simply delivering the information it wants or needs to give them.

Table 2.2 lists what patients consider the biggest priorities for improving health services based on a balance of importance (correlation to overall satisfaction) and current national performance (mean score). This measure has been dubbed the Priority Index and represents the most effective way to understand how patients would prioritize any improvement efforts. The highest priorities are areas of low performance and high importance. Again, the same issues dominate: response; communication; care and concern; and patients' unique personal, emotional, and spiritual needs. Basically, patients are saying, "If you fix anything, please fix this. This matters more to me than anything else, and it needs to get better."

The emergence of these issues as patients' biggest priorities is significant. These surveys include many measures on technical quality, process quality, safety, amenities, and environment. While patients do rate other items (e.g., meals) lower, these technical aspects of care simply do not matter as much to patients. Only once does an issue explicitly regarding amenities or physical environment appear: cheerfulness of the practice (typically interpreted by respondents as a

Table 2.1: Strongest Correlations to Patients' Loyalty

			Care Setting		
Rank	Acute Inpatient	Outpatient	Emergency Department	Medical Practice	Nursing Home
1	Response to concerns/complaints	Staff worked together	Staff cared about you as a person	Confidence in the provider	Receptiveness to your ideas
2	Special/personal needs	Response to concerns/complaints	Information about delays	Cheerfulness	Treatment of visitors
3	Sensitivity to the inconvenience caused by health problems/ hospitalization	Sensitivity to your needs	Pain control	Our sensitivity to your needs	Treated with dignity
4	Nurses keep you informed	Concern for your questions and worries	Nurses keep you informed	Concern for your questions and worries	Responsiveness to your ideas
5	Inclusion in decision making	Staff concern for your comfort	Staff keep family informed	Explanation of problem and inclusion in decision making	Explanation of your care

Table 2.2: Patients' Greatest Priorities for Health Services

			Care Setting		
Rank	Acute Inpatient	Outpatient	Emergency Department	Medical Practice	Nursing Home
1	Response to concerns/complaints	Response to concerns/complaints	Informed about delays	Our sensitivity to your needs	Responsiveness
2	Sensitivity to the inconvenience caused by health problems/hospitalization	Our sensitivity to your needs	Staff cared about you as a person	Cheerfulness	Receptive to your ideas
3	Emotional/spiritual needs	Staff worked together	Pain control	Comfort and pleasantness of the exam room	Keep you informed
4	Inclusion in decision making	Comfort of the waiting area	Nurses keep you informed	Wait time	Responsiveness to your ideas
5	Nurses keep you informed	Staff concern for your questions/worries	Wait time	Convenience of office hours	Explanation of your care

global assessment of the collective attitude of all providers and staff at the clinic). Assessments of process only appear twice: wait time. Explicit evaluation of a safety, security, or technical quality issue only appears one time: pain control in the emergency department.

When we do ask patients specifically to evaluate the safety and security of health services and the healthcare environment, what drives their assessments? The strongest drivers of patients' perceptions in these areas are information provision, sensitivity to inconvenience caused by health problems and hospitalization, response to concerns or complaints, and emotional or spiritual needs. This tells us that what makes a health services environment safe and what makes people think and feel that a health services environment is safe are two completely different things. How we are treated by those delivering the health service drives our perception of safety and security in that environment. As Press Ganey researcher and psychologist Robert Wolosin, Ph.D., (2004) concluded, "Hospitals can maximize their patients' perceptions of safety and security by globally attending to the personhood of patients."

Every year, Press Ganey researchers conduct these analyses using the past year's data to understand, at a global level, what patients want. Since 2001, every year the results have been incredibly similar. Rigorous psychometric tests, such as confirmatory factor analyses, are conducted to verify that the results are not due to the survey, methodology, or some other factor. And every year the same results resurface, placing strong emphasis on respecting personhood. No matter how the data are sliced and diced, this theme continually emerges.

Taking into consideration the research presented here and the volumes of supporting data, we can posit that the following factors constitute universal human needs that should be taken into account in the design, delivery, and management of any health service:

- responding and being sensitive to patients' unique needs;
- responding to concerns and complaints;
- emotional and spiritual needs; and
- communication quality—informing, involving, and explaining to patients as well as displaying concern and caring.

PERSONHOOD, LOYALTY, AND BREAKTHROUGH PERFORMANCE

With this understanding, we can take healthcare to the next level, beyond the Maslowian safety-at-all-costs mentality and beyond the ethics-, law-, or regulation-driven checklist approach to patient autonomy. Healthcare can deliver services that are safe, effective, timely, efficient, equitable, and patient centered not only according to managers but also according to patients—the people on the receiving end. This patient-inspired approach raises healthcare organizations to the position they deserve—not just a business that meets customer needs but one that respects and enhances the personhood of its customers.

Good to Great (Collins 2001) highlighted the importance of the hedgehog concept—a single concept that, if followed extremely well and to the virtual exclusion of almost everything else, can help a business achieve its full potential. Safety is not the hedgehog; autonomous, consumerist medicine is not the hedgehog. Personhood can be healthcare's hedgehog:

> Breakthroughs require a simple, hedgehog-like understanding of three intersecting circles: what a company can be the best in the world at, how its economics work best, and what best ignites the passions of its people. Breakthroughs happen when you get the hedgehog concept and become systematic and consistent with it (Collins 2001).

Healthcare is delivered by human beings, for human beings, to serve our most basic human needs. The more healthcare becomes a real marketplace, the greater will be the emphasis on strengthening the connection between providers and patients.

Patients' Ratings and Loyalty

When patients evaluate their relationships with health services providers, they distinguish between contentment or marginally positive satisfaction and endearing loyalty and affection. Like customers in other service industries (Hart, Heskett, and Sasser 1990), patients can exhibit a false loyalty to their providers. Even if they respect clinicians' medical expertise and technical skill, many patients do not like the way providers communicate (Arora, Singer, and Arora 2004). During the encounter, patients will not tell clinicians their true opinion of the provider's behavior. True opinions will only emerge after the fact, on surveys and, if presented with a potentially better option, in loyalty behaviors.

The strongest predictor of a patient's decision to return and bring her family members occurs when she provides the highest possible rating (e.g., Bertakis, Roter, and Putnam 1991; Press 2002). Only those patients giving the service or provider a five on a one-to-five scale can be considered truly loyal. Customers providing other ratings are flight risks. You have not won their hearts and minds; they are simply waiting for something better to come along (see Figure 2.2).

This top-box approach seeks to maximize the number of customers giving your organization a rating of five or "very good." In other words, the approach aims for consistently superlative service quality survey responses with the high rating or "top box" checked. Moving the "fair" and "good" satisfied patients into the zone of "wow" or "very good" will turn them into intensely loyal customers, leading to greater market share and achievement of financial objectives. According to Jones and Sasser (1995):

> Managers should be concerned rather than heartened if the majority of their customers fall into the satisfied (as opposed to completely satisfied) category. Most managers probably would be happy to learn that 82 percent of their customers fell into category four or five. The more appropriate reaction would be: "We have a problem. Only 48 percent of our customers are completely satisfied (scoring a five), and 52 percent are up for grabs."

The top-box approach to loyalty also drives comparative results. Table 2.3 illustrates additional consequences of the top box on percentile rank. Healthcare organizations in the top percentile ranks (91st and above) had 63 percent of patients rate them "very good,"

Figure 2.2: Patient Loyalty and Satisfaction

Loyalty and Satisfaction

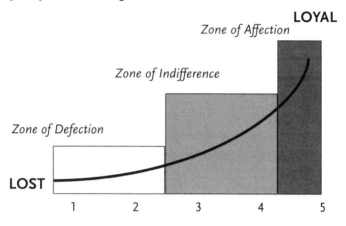

Source: Adapted from Jones and Sasser (1995).

more than twice as many as those rated simply "good." On the other hand, organizations in the bottom 10 percent had only 41 percent "very good" ratings. Healthcare organizations in the lowest decile had almost as many "good" ratings as "very good" ratings. Without benchmarking and the top-box approach, this could lead to the erroneous conclusion that patients are satisfied and loyal, when, in fact, their comparative performance is quite poor and their patients are at risk. Overall, the best performing healthcare organizations received 22 percent more "very good" responses than the worst performing organizations. This means that an additional 22 percent of their patient population are loyal to the healthcare organization and will be unlikely to defect. This kind of loyalty and positive word-of-mouth can mean a lot to the health service's financial security.

Figure 2.3, which precisely quantifies the model presented in Figure 2.2, demonstrates that a real, substantial difference exists between the healthcare services that patients evaluate poorly and those patients believe are top notch. This pattern holds true across all healthcare services as well as for patient and employee satisfaction. The mes-

Table 2.3: Analysis of Patient Satisfaction Response Category % by Percentile Rank for Inpatient Acute Care, 2004

% Difference Between

Response	90th Percentile and 10th Percentile
Very poor	2%
Poor	3%
Fair	8%
Good	9%
Very good	22%

sage: there is a quantifiable difference between mediocre healthcare organizations and those that patients believe to be exceptional.

These comparative results are important for two reasons. First, percentile ranks serve as a gauge of differentiation in service excellence. Compared to all other organizations in the United States, have you

Figure 2.3: Average percent "Very Good" Ratings by Overall Percentile, Rank

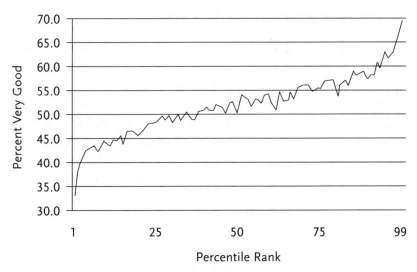

The Data Represents the Experiences of 2,170,994 Patients at 1,506 Hospitals Nationwide Between January 1 and December 31, 2004.

effectively differentiated yourself? If you provide better service quality than 90 percent of all other organizations like yours, you have a distinct competitive advantage. Second, many studies have linked patient perceptions of quality and financial objectives, particularly profit margin. In a study of 82 hospitals, a 1 percent standard deviation change in the quality score resulted in a 2 percent increase in operating margin (Harkey and Vraciu 1992). Another study of 51 hospitals ascertained that up to 30 percent of the variance in hospital profitability can be attributed to patient perceptions of the quality of care (Nelson et al. 1992). Yet more research found that a 5 percent patient dissatisfaction rate can cost a private physician $150,000 in lost revenue (Drain and Kaldenberg 1994). A recent study at Rush University Medical Center examined every factor in the Press Ganey patient survey for its impact on loyalty to determine where the biggest financial return on investment for improvement would lie. Of all factors, if patient perceptions of how well clinicians provided information moved up from ratings of three or four to ratings of four or five, the resulting increase in admissions would produce $2.3 million in additional patient revenue, or an additional $82 for each current patient (Garman, Garcia, and Hargeaves 2004).

What's Their Story? What's Your Story?

Organizations exhibiting exceptional performance in patient satisfaction and loyalty are distinguished by relentless prioritization and novel approaches to personhood. If you do not want to be average—if you want your organization to be at the top of the bell curve in meeting patients' needs—your organization must understand and address those human needs in a unique way. Being significantly better at anything is by definition different. If you do things exactly the same way as everyone else, you will probably get exactly the same results.

Understanding patients' stories

Patients are people, healthcare professionals are people, and each person is on an individual life journey. Each person has his own narrative and life story. As one person's journey derails, for a time, we become cotravelers in the healthcare encounter. As if the physical sensations of pain and illness are not enough, the person entering the foreign world of being a patient becomes enveloped by unfamiliar people, unusual machines and technology, strange sounds, never-before-experienced events, and incomprehensible processes and policies.

People do not want to be in this world; they want a return to their life journeys as they were before the illness. They want a return to wellness. They want to be and function like normal. Any person wants to regain the ability to do what she most wants to do with her life, to be what she wants to be—whatever gives her life's journey meaning and purpose and comprises her identity as a person, be that a mother, athlete, businessperson, leader, rebel, friend, teacher, film buff, or rabid sports fan.

The healthcare professional's role is to help each person recognize and come to terms with his life's journey as it has been altered. Indeed, we value medicine because it helps us understand our telos— the kind and amount of power we possess that enables us to live meaningfully within society. Maybe recovery is possible through the tribulation of therapy. Or maybe this is the start of the end of life's journey. The patient's and healthcare professional's goal is to return the patient as near as possible to the before state or help him continue on the journey after and to alleviate suffering along that journey, whatever the details of the story.

Understanding your story

It is up to you, as a leader in your organization, to imagine, envision, decide, tell, and fulfill your organization's story. Just like every person has a story, every organization has a story. If you do not envision and act to fulfill your organization's story, it will be written for you (and probably won't be as exciting or amazing as it would have been had you been proactive).

What is your organization's story right now? Be honest. Only a small minority will be truly world-class in some aspect of health services. What do you want your organization's story to be? Now that you know and understand the imperative for personhood, how will your organization systematically integrate respect for personhood into and throughout the organization?

This is the therapeutic relationship clinicians imagine being a part of before beginning medical school. Healthcare management's goal in designing a health service should be to enhance this therapeutic relationship because all outcomes—clinical, financial, satisfaction, and loyalty—flow from the encounter between the healthcare professional and the person/customer/patient in need. From this person's perspective, enhancing the therapeutic relationship includes physical, mental, spiritual, and emotional needs. These are not four different things that occur at four different times; they happen all at once, in the same encounter.

Healthcare providers are people who need to be able to do their best to serve patients. They chose a vocation in which they can devote their entire beings to helping people and serving the most fundamental human need—saving, extending, and enhancing life. This is why patient, employee, and medical staff satisfaction all correlate highly with each other in a reinforcing cycle. As leaders of healthcare organizations ask, "Who are we to our employees? What do we represent?" Envision and summarize: in one year what do you want your relationship with employees, patients, and physicians to be like? Is your organization a place that enhances their lives, stories, and journeys?

The purpose of healthcare management is to establish an appropriate environment in which the provider-patient encounter can take place. This setting must be conducive to enabling and empowering the healthcare professional and patient/customer/person to engage in an encounter in which together they build life-changing and life-affirming episodes into their personal life journeys.

Everything healthcare management does must enhance associates' ability to bring their best to serve patients' sense of personhood. Employees and physicians are the living embodiment of your organization's story, and they are the only way your health service can address and respect the personhood of patients. By evoking internal emotional responses, enhancing operations, and making employees' and medical staff's lives easier, the physical environment can support this mission.

When patients', employees', and physicians' life journeys intersect with your organization, their stories merge and blend with your organization's story. Each person in the therapeutic encounter walks away knowing and living with at least a part of someone else's story. When patients walk away from your facility, what are they taking with them?

Ask yourself: "What is my organization known for?" (List one or two things.) "In one year what will my organization be known for?" (List one or two things.) In one or two sentences define and summarize your organization's relationship with employees, physicians, and patients. What do you do better or differently than anyone else? What truly makes your organization special? And do not answer "quality." Achieving success in the competitive marketplace of the future mandates differentiation. What is your organization's story, and how does your environment support and fulfill your organization's story in the lives of patients, employees, and physicians?

The most superlative healthcare delivery organizations in the eyes of patients have a unique sense of story and deliver on it. Consider the following examples:

- Robert Wood Johnson University Hospital Hamilton's emergency department: "We respond to you in a time of need by guaranteeing that you will see a nurse in 15 minutes and a physician in 30 minutes or your emergency department fee is waived." This defines and affects everything in structuring the hospital's emergency department operations.
- Baptist Hospital System's "Healing Hospital and Radical Loving Care" initiative: (1) every single employee partner treats patients with loving care—we call this the continuous chain of caring, (2) every single leader treats staff with love and respect, (3) all hiring is done with a focus on finding people who have a Servant's Heart, (4) orientation and staff reviews are focused on a balanced evaluation of both results and values, (5) people who cannot support this approach are

respectfully removed from the organization" (Chapman 2005). This goes beyond a mission statement to ensuring that it is practiced every day by every associate.

- Planetree: "Our mission is to help hospitals provide more personalized, humanistic, patient centered health care in a healing environment; to empower individuals to be actively involved in decisions affecting their care and well-being through access to information and education; and to provide leadership to improve the health of the communities served." Planetree differentiates themselves by creating a total operational and service environment designed to promote patient and family involvement in their care.
- Eden Alternative: "We must teach ourselves to see the environments as habitats for human beings rather than facilities for the frail and elderly. We must learn what Mother Nature has to teach us about the creation of vibrant, vigorous habitats. The Eden Alternative™ (2005) shows us how companion animals, the opportunity to give meaningful care to other living creatures, and the variety and spontaneity that mark an enlivened environment can succeed where pills and therapies fail." Eden Alternative redefined the basic idea of nursing homes and long-term care. "Vibrant, vigorous habitats," "meaningful care," and "variety...spontaneity...enlivene environment" evoke different imagery, imagery reinforced in the total facility design (Eden 2005).

Everything in your organization flows into the same message, story, myth, and theme. Think about it this way: if someone wanted to make a movie about your organization, what would the plot be? What would be the lessons learned by all of the characters? How would the characters' lives change? Everything aligns to tell, reinforce, perform, and deliver your story. How does your environment tell your story? Everything speaks. What are the clues your environment gives its customers? What symbols are you using to communicate your organization's story and the integration of patients' stories? How does your environment communicate respect for personhood? Is the environment saying

- you are safe here;
- we are trustworthy;
- it is a joy and pleasure to serve you in this time of need;
- we connect with you on a spiritual and emotional level;
- we respect your personhood;
- we respond to your needs;
- we strengthen your family;
- we are here for you;
- we care for you; and
- we love you?

CONCLUSION

Personhood is defined by the fulfillment of human needs. Patients are people who need health services to be able to fulfill their human needs. Fundamentally, healthcare organizations are in the business of helping people achieve personhood. The most successful health services and products on the market recognize and speak to the personhood of the patient. Technical care for the patienthood is always expected, but the human being fundamentally desires care for her unique personhood.

All of the data ultimately can be understood as a call to respect personhood by serving the unique needs of the individual. It becomes clear that the similarities in these results outweigh the differences. The common theme is that the better organizations are at responding to personhood, the more satisfied people are and the more likely they will be to recommend and return to the health services of these organizations. This represents a universal theme, consistently reappearing across every way we have cut the data. Cumulatively, respect for personhood represents the definitive answer to the question, "What do patients want?

Different individuals—of different cultures, religions, and ages; with different illnesses, physical and mental functioning, and past experiences; and possessed by different hopes and dreams—will all hold different needs for achieving personhood. Healthcare executives cannot sit in their offices and design a service that enables personhood because personhood is different for every person. The healthcare manager must set the stage, design the environment, provide the tools, and enable the clinician through support and training to adaptively attend to helping patients become persons through the fulfillment of their human needs.

ACKNOWLEDGMENTS

We acknowledge the contributions of Laura Vercler, Kelly Leddy, and Kimberly McCaffrey, who conducted research analyses to support these findings.

NOTE

1. For enthralling accounts of the human need for positive emotion, humor, laughter, love, and hope, see Victor Frankl's (1984) *Man's Search for Meaning* or Norman Cousins's (1979) *Anatomy of an Illness as Perceived by the Patient.*

REFERENCES

Arora, R., J. Singer, and A. Arora. 2004. "Influence of Key Variables on the Patient's Choice of a Physician." *Quality Management in Health Care* 13 (3): 166–73.

Ashley, B., and K. O'Rourke. 2002. *Ethics of Health Care.* Washington, DC: Georgetown University Press.

Bertakis, K., D. Roter, and S. Putnam. 1991. "The Relationship of Physician Medical Interview Style to Patient Satisfaction." *Journal of Family Practice* 32 (2): 175–81.

Chapman, E. 2005. *Radical Loving Care.* Fourth Printing. Nashville, TN: Baptist Healing Hospital Trust.

Collins, J. 2001. *Good to Great: Why Some Companies Make the Leap . . . And Others Don't.* New York: HarperCollins.

Cousins, N. 1979. *Anatomy of an Illness as Perceived by the Patient.* New York: Bantam Books.

Drain, M., and D. Kaldenberg. 1994. "Building Patient Loyalty and Trust: The Role of Patient Satisfaction." *Group Practice Journal* 48 (9): 32–35.

Eden Alternative. 2005. "What is Eden?" [Online information; retrieved 08/22/05.] www.edenalticom/about.htm.

Frankl, V. 1984. *Man's Search for Meaning.* New York: Simon & Schuster.

Garman, A, J. Garcia, and M. Hargeaves. 2004. "Patient Satisfaction as a Predictor of Return-to-Provider Behavior: Analysis and Assessment of Financial Implications." *Quality Management in Health Care* 13 (1): 75–80.

Harkey, J., and R. Vraciu. 1992. "Quality of Health Care and Financial Performance: Is there a Link?" *Health Care Management Review* 17 (4): 55–63.

Hart, C., J. Heskett, and W. Sasser, Jr. 1990. "Zero Defections: Quality Comes to Services." *Harvard Business Review* 68 (5): 105–11.

Hastie, R., and R. Dawes. 2001. *Rational Choice in an Uncertain World: The Psychology of Judgment and Decision Making.* Thousand Oaks, CA: Sage Publications.

Institute of Medicine. 2001. *Crossing the Quality Chasm: A New Health System for the 21st Century.* Washington, DC: National Academies Press.

Jones, T., and W. Sasser, Jr. 1995. "Why Satisfied Customers Defect." *Harvard Business Review* 73 (6):88–99.

Maslow, A. 1987. *Motivation and Personality, 3rd Edition.* New York: Harper & Row.

Nelson, E., R. Rust, A. Zahorik, R. Rose, P. Batalden, and B. Siemanski. 1992. "Do Patient Perceptions of Quality Relate to Hospital Financial Performance?" *Journal of Health Care Marketing* 12 (4): 6–13.

Press, I. 2002. *Patient Satisfaction: Defining, Measuring, and Improving the Experience of Care.* Chicago: Health Administration Press.

Pascal, B. 1941. *Penses* [1669]. New York: Modern Library.

Robert Wood Johnson University Hospital Hamilton. 2005. "Emergency Services." [Online article; retrieved 08/22/05.] www.rwjhamilton.org/medserv.emerg.asp.

Wolosin, R. 2004. "Patients' Perceptions of Safety in U.S. Hospitals." Presentation at the Annual Research Meeting of the Academy of Health, San Diego, California. June 6–8.

CHAPTER 3

The Environment's Impact on Stress

Roger S. Ulrich, Ph.D.; Craig Zimring, Ph.D.;
Xiaobo Quan, and Anjali Joseph

UNDERSTANDING STRESS IS fundamental to understanding how physical healthcare environments affect outcomes (Ulrich 1991). Much research has demonstrated that hospitalized patients experience considerable stress. Examples of stressful aspects of hospitalization include painful medical procedures, fear about impending surgery, reduced physical capabilities, loss of control, depersonalization through bureaucratic processing, and disruption of social relationships. Many stressers are unavoidable aspects of illness and medical procedures, whereas others stem from the healthcare organizational culture. Additional major stress is produced by poorly designed physical environments that deny privacy, are noisy, make wayfinding difficult, do not allow patients to see out of windows, or hinder the presence of family (Ulrich 1991).

In addition to affecting patients, stress is a major problem for families of patients and for staff such as nurses. Healthcare occupations are stressful because they usually involve lack of control, overload from escalating work demands, rotating shifts, and other stressful events such as patient death. Further contributing to employee stress are poorly designed healthcare workplaces that are noisy, increase fatigue, hinder patient care activities, and lack adequate employee lounges or respite areas.

For patients stress is an important medical outcome in itself and substantially influences many other types of outcomes (Cohen, Tyrrell, and Smith 1991; Ulrich 1999). These widespread negative effects are related to psychological, physiological, neuroendocrine, and behavioral manifestations of stress (Gatchel, Baum, and Krantz 1989). The psychological component includes worrisome thoughts, a sense of helplessness, and feelings of fear or sadness. Physiological manifestations involve changes in bodily system activity levels—for example, higher blood pressure, heart rate, and muscle tension. The neuroendocrine component generates hormones and a natural steroid, cortisol, that influence the heart and other major organs. Behavioral manifestations of stress include passivity, social withdrawal, verbal outbursts, sleeplessness, and noncompliance with medical regimens (Ulrich 1991, 1999).

Stress responses mobilize a person for dealing with a taxing or threatening situation, but they consume energy and increase fatigue. Much research also has demonstrated that stress responses, via their effects in heightening neuroendocrine activity and activating the central nervous system, suppress immune system functioning (Kiecolt-Glaser et al. 1987). Stress-related immune impairment decreases resistance to infection and slows or worsens recovery outcomes. When patients are stressed, for example, wounds heal more slowly (Kiecolt-Glaser et al. 1995).

The foregoing indicates strong grounds for contending that outcomes will be worsened if healthcare facilities have features or characteristics that are in themselves stressers. Conversely, healthcare environments should foster improved outcomes if they are designed to minimize stressers such as noise and promote exposure to physical features and social situations that have stress-reducing influences (Ulrich 1991).

Portions of this chapter are based on the results of a literature review conducted for The Center for Health Design (The Center) and funded by the Robert Wood Johnson Foundation (Ulrich et al. 2004). The review identified more than 350 rigorous scientific studies relevant to understanding how physical healthcare environments affect patient stress and other outcomes.

HOSPITAL NOISE

Noise Levels and Sources

A large body of rigorous research, running to more than 135 published studies, has focused on noise in hospitals and other healthcare buildings. This work has unequivocally documented that hospitals are loud environments, with noise levels far exceeding World Health Organization (WHO) guideline values. WHO guidelines specify 35 decibels (dB) or less for continuous background noise in patient rooms, with nighttime peaks not to exceed 40 dB (Berglund, Lindvall, and Schwela 1999). Hospital background noise levels commonly are in the range of 45 to 68 dB, with peaks frequently exceeding 80 to 90 dB (Allaouchiche et al. 2002; Hilton 1985; Meyer et al. 1994; Robertson, Cooper-Peel, and Vos 1998). Staff voices and medical equipment commonly produce 70 to 75 dB measured at the patient's head. Noises from alarms, bedrails moved up and down, nurse shift changes, and equipment such as portable x-ray machines exceed 90 dB, similar to walking next to a highway when a large truck passes.

Hospitals are excessively noisy because noise sources are unnecessarily numerous and loud, and many environmental surfaces (floors, ceilings, walls) are hard and sound reflecting, enabling noise to echo, linger, and propagate over large areas and into patient rooms (Ulrich, Lawson, and Martinez 2003). Examples of commonly documented noise sources include telephones, trolleys, ice machines, paging systems, staff voices, and roommates.

Single- Versus Multi-Bed Rooms

Noise is a much greater problem in multi- than single-bed rooms. Most noise in multi-bed rooms is linked to the presence of roommates (staff caring for other patients, equipment, sliding bedrails, doors closing, visitors, patients crying out or coughing) (Southwell and Wistow 1995; Yinnon et al. 1992). Furthermore, the patient in a multi-bed room has no control over noises linked to other patients.

Uncontrollable noise is more likely to be stressful than controllable noise (Parsons and Hartig 2000).

The great advantage of single-bed rooms compared to multi-bed rooms is underscored by Press Ganey national satisfaction data showing that U.S. patients in single rooms are vastly more satisfied with noise levels in and around their rooms (Press Ganey 2003). Press Ganey obtained data for 2.1 million patients in 1,462 facilities during 2003 and showed that the pattern of much higher satisfaction with respect to noise levels for patients in single-bed rooms held across all patient categories, ages and genders, and facility sizes and types. Satisfaction with noise level was 11 percent higher on average for patients in single rooms compared to those with a roommate, a large difference considering that it can be difficult for hospitals to increase satisfaction scores by even 2 or 3 percentage points.

Effects of Noise on Patient and Staff Outcomes

A large body of research has shown that noise worsens patient outcomes. As would be expected, noise is a major cause of awakenings, sleep loss, and fragmentation (Parthasarathy and Tobin 2004; Topf and Davis 1993; Yinnon et al. 1992). Research that monitored brain electrical activity suggests that even low-decibel noise (38 dB) fragments and worsens sleep, especially when it occurs in patient rooms with poor acoustical conditions (sound-reflecting ceilings) (Berg 2001).

In addition to reducing sleep quality, noise elevates physiological stress in adult patients as indicated by increased blood pressure and heart rate (Blomkvist et al. 2005). A study of a coronary intensive care unit found that patients with acute myocardial infarction were more stressed and had a higher frequency of rehospitalization following discharge if they had experienced comparatively noisy, poor acoustical conditions during their hospital stays (Hagerman et al. 2005). In the same study upgrading the acoustical characteristics of the coronary intensive care unit by changing from sound-reflecting ceiling tile to sound-absorbing tiles decreased noise, improved sleep, and reduced stress and incidence of rehospitalization.

In addition to these studies documenting negative effects on adult patients, other research has revealed that noise degrades outcomes for infants in neonatal intensive care units (NICUs). Higher noise in NICUs worsens infant sleep and elevates blood pressure, heart rate, and respiration (Slevin et al. 2000). Furthermore, noise in NICUs decreases oxygen saturation in infants, thereby increasing the need for oxygen support therapy (Zahr and de Traversay 1995).

The body of noise research pertinent to staff is smaller than that for patients, and more studies focusing on healthcare workers are needed. Nevertheless, convincing evidence already exists that higher noise levels engender stress and annoyance among healthcare workers and are associated with emotional exhaustion and burnout (Bayo, Garcia, and Garcia 1995; Topf and Dillon 1988). Blomkvist and colleagues (2005) studied the effects of higher versus lower noise conditions over a period of months on nurses in a coronary intensive care unit. During periods with less noise, speech intelligibility increased, quality of patient care improved, workplace social support among staff was better, and nurses perceived their work demands as lessened.

Noise-Reduction Measures

It is clear from the foregoing discussion that healthcare buildings are far too noisy and that noise in combination with poor acoustical surfaces and conditions substantially worsens patient and staff outcomes. New building designs accordingly should place high priority on creating much quieter environments. Fortunately, highly effective design strategies are available for quieting hospitals and other healthcare settings.

The most important design measure for reducing noise for inpatients is to provide single-bed rooms. Another important and proven environmental intervention is to install high-performance sound-absorbing ceiling tiles that reduce echoing or reverberation and sharply diminish noise propagation (Blomkvist et al. 2005). A third key component of quieting facilities is to eliminate noise sources— for example, by replacing overhead paging with a noiseless system and insulating ice machines and pneumatic tubes. It should be mentioned that research on the impact of organizational changes or interventions for reducing noise (establishing quiet hours, educating staff to speak quietly) suggests that such approaches are much less effective than design or environmental interventions (Gast and Baker 1989; Walder et al. 2000). The key to achieving a quiet healthcare building is found mainly in appropriate design of the physical environment, not in modifying organizational culture or staff behavior.

SPATIAL DISORIENTATION

Wayfinding or navigation problems in hospitals are stressful and costly and negatively affect outpatients and visitors, who are often unfamiliar with the building and otherwise stressed and disoriented. A study conducted at a major 604-bed tertiary hospital in 1990 found that the annual cost of an inadequate wayfinding system was more than $220,000, or $448 per bed per year. Much of this cost stemmed from time consumed giving directions by healthcare workers other than information staff, which occupied more than 4,500 staff hours, the equivalent of more than two full-time positions (Zimring 1990).

While almost all hospitals strongly feel the problems associated with a complicated large building and poor wayfinding system, it is usually difficult and ineffective to tackle this problem with a piecemeal approach. A wayfinding system, as the name implies, is not just about better signage or colored lines on floors. Rather, hospitals are seeking to provide integrated systems that include coordinated elements such as visible and easy-to-understand signs and numbers; clear and consistent verbal directions and paper, mailed, and electronic information; and a physical setting that offers cues to help people find their way (Carpman and Grant 1993). An effective wayfinding system includes four main components that work at different levels: (1) administrative and procedural information, (2) external building cues, (3) local information, and (4) global structure.

Administrative and Procedural Information

Mailed maps, electronic information available on the Internet and at kiosks, and verbal directions are organizational strategies aimed at providing key information to patients to prepare them for their hospital visits. These are not dealt with in this review.

External Building Cues

Signs and cues that lead to the hospital or clinic, especially the parking lot, need to be considered carefully, as they are the first point of patient contact with the building (Carpman, Grant, and Simmons 1985). For example, Carpman, Grant, and Simmons conducted a video simulation study to assess the relative role of signs and seeing a destination. The hospital wished to direct most traffic to a parking structure rather than a drop-off lane. When prospective visitors viewed a simulated video showing a design alternative that allowed arriving drivers to see the main pavilion with the drop-off lane, 37 percent of the respondents said they would turn into the drop circle when they could see the entry to the garage, ignoring the signs. As a consequence the hospital chose to redesign the entry.

Local Information

Once patients find their way to the building from the parking lot, they are faced with the task of identifying the destination. Informational handouts, information desks, you-are-here maps, directories, and signage along the way are critical wayfinding aids (Carpman, Grant, and Simmons 1983–84; Levine, Marchon, and Hanley 1984; Nelson-Shulman 1983–84; Wright, Hull, and Lickorish 1993). Using an experimental research design, investigators found that patients who had the benefit of an information system (welcome sign, hospital information booklet, patient letter, orientation aids) upon reaching the admitting area were more self-reliant and made fewer demands on staff. In contrast, uninformed patients rated the hospital less favorably and had higher heart rates (Nelson-Shulman 1983–84).

Information provided in you-are-here maps can be useful. However, for ease of use such maps should be oriented so that the top signifies the direction of movement. When the maps are aligned in directions other than the forward position, people take much longer to find their destinations and are less accurate in their navigation (Levine, Marchon, and Hanley 1984). Another study found that people who used signs found their destinations faster than those who only used maps (Butler et al. 1993). However, those who were given a combination of handheld maps and wall signs reached their destinations more often than those who just used wall signs (Wright, Hull, and Lickorish 1993).

It is critical to design signage systems with logical room numbering and comprehensible nomenclature for departments (Carpman and Grant 1993; Carpman, Grant, and Simmons 1984). For example, inpatients, outpatients, and visitors to a hospital preferred simple terms such as "walkway" or "general hospital" over more complex or less familiar terms such as "overhead link," "medical pavilion," or "health sciences complex."

Contrary to the belief that fewer signs in hospital hallways mean less clutter and hence less confusion, an experimental study in a hospital found that patients who had access to a greater number of signs along the way to their destinations were faster, less hesitant, asked for directions less often, and reported lower levels of stress (Carpman, Grant, and Simmons 1984). Based on these findings, the authors suggested that directional signs should be placed at or before every major intersection, at major destinations, and where a single environmental cue or series of such cues (e.g., change in flooring material) conveys the message that the individual is moving from one area into another. If there are no key decision points along a route, signs should be placed approximately every 150 to 250 feet.

Global Structure

In addition to local properties of the spaces through which people move, there are specific characteristics of the overall structure of the system of rooms and corridors that affect the paths people take (Haq and Zimring 2003; Peponis, Zimring, and Choi 1990). People tend to move toward spaces and through corridors that are more accessible from a greater number of spaces. Based on observations of search patterns of study participants in a hospital and data from objective measurements that quantify spatial characteristics, researchers found that participants tended to move along more integrated routes— routes that are on average more accessible because they are fewer turns away from all other routes in the hospital. Their findings suggest that it may be important to identify such integrated routes in the plan when designing or locating important facilities and key points such as the entrance (Peponis, Zimring, and Choi 1990).

The research supports the value of a systems approach to wayfinding. Wayfinding continues to be a pervasive problem in hospitals because it is insufficient to consider or implement one or two components separately. Even well-designed signs are likely to be ineffective in a building that is highly complicated and does not provide simple cues that enable natural movement. While at least 17 studies have examined wayfinding in hospitals and other buildings (e.g., Christensen 1979; Grover 1971; Ortega-Andeane and Urbina-Soria 1988; Schneider and Taylor 1999), it has proven difficult for investigators to isolate single influences of design on wayfinding performance or of wayfinding on outpatient or visitor stress. The problem is exacerbated by the fact that most hospitals have existing complex buildings on which they try to superimpose a signage system to make things work. This strategy is ineffective in most cases.

There are some strong studies that deal, for example, with designing better signage, optimal spacing and location of signage, or types of information that are most effective in wayfinding. Other studies at the global level have looked at the properties of building layout that facilitate or impede movement. It is essential that these different pieces of information come together while designing new hospitals, where there is opportunity to develop an effective wayfinding system at multiple levels. Additional studies are needed to ascertain the magnitude of stress that wayfinding problems produce in outpatients and family and possible negative aftereffects evident in clinical outcomes.

ACCESS TO NATURE AND POSITIVE DISTRACTION

Positive distractions are a small category of environmental conditions, features, and contents (e.g., water) that research has shown effectively reduce stress. Distractions used frequently in healthcare settings include companion animals such as dogs or cats, gardening, art with emotionally appropriate subject matter, and especially nature (Frumpkin 2001; Ulrich 1991). The focus here will be mainly on the last of these, nature. Music also is widely used as a distraction in healthcare situations, but the large literature on music is not surveyed here.

Stress-Reducing Effects of Viewing Nature

The notion that certain types of nature settings reduce stress is underpinned partly by findings from a score of scientific studies on populations other than healthcare patients. This research has convincingly demonstrated that visual exposure to real or simulated views of nature produces substantial emotional or psychological and physiological recovery from stress within three to five minutes at most, or as quickly as 20 seconds in some bodily systems (Parsons and Hartig 2000; Ulrich 1999; Ulrich 1991; Van den Berg, Koole, and Van der Wulp 2003). Investigators have reliably found that stress-reducing or restorative effects of looking at nature are manifested as a collection of positive changes characterized by heightened positive feelings, reduced negative emotions such as fear or anger, and changes in physiological systems indicating lower stress mobilization (cardiovascular, electrocortical, neuroendocrine, musculoskeletal) (Parsons and Hartig 2000; Ulrich 1991). Although viewing most nature settings reduces stress, considerable evidence suggests that many urban or built scenes (streets, parking lots, windowless rooms, buildings without nature) are ineffective in fostering recuperation and may exacerbate stress (Ulrich 1991; Van den Berg, Koole, and Van der Wulp 2003).

In findings that closely parallel those obtained for stressed non-patient groups, research in healthcare settings has shown that exposure to nature can quickly and effectively lower stress. For example, a prospective controlled experiment found that stressed blood donors in a waiting room had lower blood pressure and pulse rates on days when a wall-mounted television displayed a nature videotape compared to days when the television showed daytime television programs such as game or talk shows (Ulrich, Simons, and Miles 2003). A study of patients with late-stage dementia suggested that adding color nature pictures and recorded nature sounds (birds, babbling brook) to a shower room reduced stress and agitated aggressive behavior (hitting, biting, kicking) (Whall et al. 1997).

Pain-Reducing Effects of Viewing Nature

Several strong studies using experimental or quasiexperimental designs have shown convincingly that, apart from reducing stress, viewing nature alleviates patient pain. In explaining why exposure to nature should reduce pain most investigators have referred to distraction/pain theory. According to distraction theory humans have a limited amount of available conscious attention. In the case of patients, pain requires conscious attention and draws heavily on the limited amount available. If patients become engrossed in or are diverted by a pleasant distraction such as a nature scene, they will have less conscious attention to allocate to pain and accordingly will subjectively experience less pain (Hoffman et al. 2000; McCaul and Malott 1984).

Other authors have proposed a variant of this explanation by integrating distraction theory with the gate-control theory of pain. In gate theory the transmission of nerve impulses through the spinal cord to the brain is modulated by spinal mechanisms that act like a gate. Environmental distraction can close the gate and prevent or reduce the transmission of pain nerve impulses, thereby inhibiting pain messages from reaching the brain (Melzack and Wall 1965; Tse et al. 2002).

Several studies indicate that nature distraction can produce substantial and clinically important pain mitigation. Patients recovering from abdominal surgery needed far fewer potent narcotic pain doses and had better emotional well-being and shorter hospital stays if they had bedside windows with a nature view (trees) than if their windows overlooked a brick wall (Ulrich 1984). A study of burn patients suffering intense pain revealed that distraction with a videotape of scenic nature (waterfalls, forest, flowers, ocean) during burn-dressing changes markedly lowered both pain intensity and anxiety or stress (Miller, Hickman, and Lemasters 1992). A randomized prospective study of adults undergoing a painful bronchoscopy procedure showed that patients experienced less pain if they were assigned to look at a ceiling-mounted nature scene rather than a blank ceiling control condition (Diette et al. 2003). Another well-controlled experiment found that volunteers in a hospital had a significantly higher threshold for detecting pain and much greater pain tolerance when they viewed a nature videotape in contrast to looking at a blank screen (Tse et al. 2002). In addition, studies have used virtual-reality nature displays (e.g., walk through a forest with bird sounds) to reduce stress, discomfort, and symptomatic distress in groups such as women with cancer (Schneider et al. 2004).

Gardens for Improving Outcomes

Gardens in healthcare settings provide calming or stress-reducing views and, if properly designed, mitigate stress and improve outcomes through a number of other established mechanisms or pathways. For example, well-designed gardens can create enticing opportunities for patients to engage in physical activity or movement or provide pleasant spaces for sitting with family and engaging in healthful social interaction and support (Ulrich 1999). Findings from postoccupancy evaluations indicate that patients and family members who use gardens in hospitals or clinics report reduced stress and enhanced emotional well-being (Cooper-Marcus and Barnes 1995; Sherman et al. forthcoming; Whitehouse et al. 2001).

These investigations further suggest that healthcare gardens can increase patient and family satisfaction with overall quality of care. Evidence also suggests that gardens tend to be especially effective in alleviating stress in adult patients and family members when they contain green or relatively verdant foliage, nonturbulent water, grassy spaces with trees or large shrubs and some spatial openness, and compatible pleasant nature sounds (breezes, water, birds) (Cooper-

Marcus and Barnes 1995; Ulrich 1999). Sherman and colleagues (forthcoming) reported that successful gardens for pediatric facilities contained prominent nature; features that permitted parents or adults to sit, socialize, or passively relax; and features for children that enabled active play and engagement.

Benefits for Healthcare Workers

Given the well-documented problems of staff stress, erosion of job satisfaction, high turnover, and shortages of nurses and other clinicians, the growing evidence indicating that nature and gardens reduce employee stress, increase job satisfaction, and may foster recruitment and retention of qualified personnel is noteworthy (Cooper-Marcus and Barnes 1995; Sherman et al. forthcoming; Whitehouse et al. 2001). Other findings relevant to healthcare workers have come from research on stressed employees in nonhealthcare workplaces. For example, a study of 100 European white- and blue-collar employees in different nonhealthcare work settings found that window views of nature buffered job stress and enhanced health-related well-being (Leather et al. 1998). In another investigation office workers with a window view of nature reported lower frustration and higher life satisfaction and overall health (Kaplan 1993).

Art in Healthcare Environments

Some artists and designers may assume that nearly all paintings and other visual art in healthcare environments are positive distractions that reduce stress and foster improved outcomes (Ulrich 1991; Ulrich and Gilpin 2003). In reality, however, the subject matter and style of visual artwork vary enormously, and much art is emotionally challenging, ambiguous, or provocative. It should be expected that certain emotionally positive art subject matter or styles will tend to have beneficial effects on patients, whereas others could be stressful and worsen outcomes (Ulrich 1991; Ulrich and Gilpin 2003). In this regard evidence is increasing that abstract, ambiguous, or other emotionally inappropriate images elicit widespread dislike and often aggravate patient stress (Ulrich 1991; Ulrich and Gilpin 2003; Ulrich, Lundén, and Eltinge 1993). Those selecting artwork should exercise caution before choosing to display abstract, emotionally negative, or surreal art in spaces where stress is a problem.

A limited amount of research on art in healthcare settings has yielded findings that parallel those from the nature studies described above. Carpman and Grant (1993) obtained art preference data from a diverse sample of 300 inpatients and found consistently high preference for representational nature images but strong dislike for abstract art. Hathorn and Ulrich likewise reported that both African Americans and Caucasians preferred representational images of nature scenes and rural landscapes. Both African Americans and Caucasians also deemed art as suitable for patient rooms if it depicted persons who displayed emotionally positive facial expressions and caring or friendly gestures and body language in nature spaces such as gardens (Ulrich and Gilpin 2003).

Also, there is evidence that representational nature art or pictures reduce stress and pain in a manner similar to the effects of real nature views. For example, heart surgery patients who were assigned a picture showing a lake and trees experienced less stress and anxiety and required fewer doses of strong pain drugs than similar patients assigned to a control group with no picture (Ulrich, Lundén, and Eltinge 1993). In the same study, however, patients assigned an abstract picture were significantly more stressed than the control group. Heerwagen (1990) found that patients in a dental clinic were less stressed on days when a large nature mural was hung on a wall of the waiting room compared to days when the wall was blank. Overall, findings support the notion that the evidence-based selection of nature art and other emotionally appropriate images contributes an important stress-reducing dimension to healthcare environments.

LIGHT EXPOSURE

Reduced Depression, Stress, and Pain

Questionnaire studies across a variety of environments (healthcare buildings, workplaces, classrooms) have found that people, including

hospitalized patients, prefer and value window views of nature illumi-
nated by clear light conditions or sunlight rather than shade or cloudy
conditions (Leather et al. 1998; Verderber 1986). Importantly, several
strong studies indicate that the significance of exposure to light—both
natural daylight and artificial light—extends far beyond preference to
include positive effects on outcomes such as sleep quality, depression,
agitation, and length of stay. A study of elderly patients with dementia found that two ten-day periods of exposure to bright morning light
reduced agitation. The same patients became significantly more agitated on nontreatment days (Lovell, Ancoli-Israel, and Gevirtz 1995).
There is also good evidence that exposure to bright light improves sleep
and circadian rhythms in elderly and other adult patients.

For young infants in NICUs, research suggests that light levels
should be altered each day to reinforce the natural diurnal variation
(Shepley 2004). Using light modulations to help synchronize infants'
circadian rhythms with those of their mothers improves sleep and
weight gain (Brandon, Holditch-Davis, and Belyea 2002).

Findings from at least 11 rigorous investigations support the conclusion that higher levels of light exposure, compared to lower levels, are effective in reducing depression among adult patients
hospitalized with severe depression and among those with bipolar
disorder and seasonal affective disorder. Several of these studies also
suggest that exposure to morning light often is more effective than
evening light in reducing depression (Benedetti et al. 2001; Terman
et al. 2001). For example, a well-controlled study that compared the
effects of morning and evening light on patients with winter depression found that morning light was twice as effective as evening light
in improving their conditions (Lewy et al. 1998). Benedetti and colleagues (2001) found that adult patients hospitalized for bipolar
depression had substantially shorter stays if they were assigned to
east-facing rooms with high levels of morning sunlight. In the same
study similar patients required longer periods of inpatient care if
they were in rooms on more shaded sides of the same building. In
a similar vein Beauchemin and Hays (1996) found that patients hospitalized for severe depression in a Canadian facility had markedly
shorter stays if they were assigned to a sunny rather than a dim,
shaded room.

It has been speculated that such depression-alleviating influences of higher levels of daylight or sunshine may explain the finding from another study that mortality of myocardial infarction patients in a Canadian hospital was lower if they were assigned to intensive care rooms having higher daylight and sun exposure rather than to north-facing shaded rooms (Beauchemin and Hays 1998).

A strong prospective study examined whether the amount of sunlight in hospital rooms influences patients' psychosocial health and intake of pain drugs (Walch et al. 2005). The researchers theorized that higher sunlight exposure would improve mood and reduce pain intensity by influencing levels of serotonin, a neurotransmitter known to inhibit pain pathways. Patients undergoing cervical and lumbar spinal surgeries were admitted postoperatively to the bright or shaded, dim side of an inpatient surgical ward. Compared to patients in the dim rooms, those in the bright rooms were exposed to 46 percent higher intensity sunlight on average, reported less stress and pain, took 22 percent less analgesic medication, and had 21 percent lower medication costs (Walch et al. 2005).

Implications for Healthcare Architecture and Site Planning

In the aforementioned pain study, heightened pain and other worsened outcomes apparently came about because an adjacent building had been constructed approximately 25 meters away, blocking sunlight exposure to patient rooms on one side of the surgical ward (Walch et al. 2005). This point underscores the importance of giving careful consideration to building orientation and site planning in new projects. The mounting scientific evidence linking higher daylight or sun exposure to improved outcomes implies that site plans should be avoided where some buildings block light from others. Another implication is that deep-plan healthcare buildings, with a large proportion of windowless rooms, may tend to worsen patient and staff stress and other outcomes.

Architectural form and orientation that enable exposure to morning sunlight should be an important consideration for wards containing patient categories known to experience depression. Another clear implication is that architectural solutions that permit little natural daylight in patient rooms should be avoided. A hypothetical example would be a hospital having patient room windows looking out into a roofed atrium with few skylights and little natural light. In this example patient deprivation of natural light exposure could be extreme if windows were tinted to prevent users of the atrium from looking into patient rooms and violating privacy.

SOCIAL SUPPORT

There is extensive evidence that social support provided to patients by family and close friends has important benefits in terms of reducing stress and improving other outcomes. Social support includes emotional support or caring derived through interpersonal relationships and tangible assistance from others. Many studies across varied patient categories spanning acute and chronic illness have indicated that social support improves, for example, recovery outcomes in myocardial infarction patients and emotional well-being and quality of life in late-stage cancer patients. The presence of a friend in a stressful situation has been shown to reduce cardiovascular reactivity (Uchino and Garvey 1997).

Despite this large body of research, there exists a shortage of studies that have directly examined whether healthcare environments that increase levels of social interaction actually promote better outcomes. The evidence showing benefits of social support across other health contexts is so convincing, however, that it seems justified to suggest that healthcare design strategies that foster social support should tend to lower stress and improve other outcomes (Ulrich 1991).

A moderate amount of research has examined how the design of healthcare environments facilitates or hinders social support for patients. Several rigorous studies focusing mainly on mental health facilities and nursing homes have demonstrated that levels of social interaction—and presumably beneficial social support—can be substantially increased by providing waiting rooms, lounges, and day rooms with comfortable and movable (not fixed) furniture arranged in small, flexible groupings. By contrast, the common practice of arranging fixed side-by-side seating along room walls strongly inhibits social interaction (Holahan 1972). A few well-designed studies in nursing homes and mental health wards have shown that appropriate arrangement of movable chairs around small rather than large dining tables increases social interaction and improves eating behaviors in clinically important ways such as increasing the amount of food consumed by geriatric patients (Melin and Gotestam 1981). Harris (2000) suggested that family and friends made longer visits to long-stay rehabilitation patients when patient rooms were carpeted rather than covered with vinyl flooring. It should be noted that when properly designed, installed, and maintained, evidence suggests that carpeting does not pose an increased risk of infection in healthcare setting, except in those areas that might be more susceptible to spills (i.e., cleaning rooms, utility rooms, and around sinks).

A great deal of evidence indicates that single-bed rooms are far better than multi-bed rooms for supporting the presence of family and friends. A clear advantage of single rooms stems from the fact that they provide more space and furniture per patient for accommodating visitors than multi-bed rooms. Compared to singles, multi-bed rooms greatly diminish privacy for patient-family interactions and are more likely to have restricted visiting hours. Some findings suggest that open-bay multi-bed rooms actually deter family presence (Sallstrom, Sandman, and Norberg 1987). Nurses' perceptions echo the superior patient satisfaction with single rooms demonstrated in the Press Ganey (2003) study discussed earlier in the chapter. A survey in four West-Coast hospitals that each had a mix of one- and two-bed rooms found that nurses gave consistently high ratings to singles for accommodating family and friends but accorded much lower scores to double rooms (Chaudhury, Mahmood, and Valente 2003).

Do patients sharing a multi-bed room provide each other with stress-reducing social support? Findings from several studies indicate that in the majority of cases the presence of a roommate is a source of stress rather than restoration. Roommates often are linked to multiple stressers—for example, a roommate who is unfriendly, seriously ill, or has too many visitors (Van der Ploeg 1988; Volicer, Isenberg, and Burns 1977). In addition to the noise considerations described in an earlier section, loss of privacy is another major stresser associated with roommates. In this regard findings from the Press Ganey satisfaction data cited earlier leave no doubt that patients in single-bed rooms, compared to those with a roommate, are consistently much more satisfied with concern for their privacy.

CONCLUSION

There is a strong and extensive body of scientific research relevant to the evidence-based design of healthcare environments that effectively reduce patient stress and improve other outcomes. High noise level is a pervasive stresser in healthcare buildings that substantially worsens patient and staff outcomes. Proven design measures for creating much quieter facilities include eliminating noise sources, installing high-performance sound-absorbing ceiling tiles, and providing single-bed rooms. Adopting a systems approach to wayfinding—combining external building cues, information sources such as you-are-here maps, numerous clear signs, and other measures—can alleviate stressful and costly navigation problems. Providing views of nature, access to gardens, and exposure to emotionally appropriate art can be effective for reducing stress and pain. Careful attention to building design, orientation, and site planning can ensure patient exposure to higher levels of natural light that reduce depression and stress, mitigate pain, and foster shorter inpatient stays. Providing single-bed rooms and waiting rooms with comfortable, movable seating facilitates the presence of family and friends who supply patients with stress-reducing social support. A theme running through much of the research is the importance of providing single-bed patient rooms for reducing stress, improving other outcomes, and markedly increasing patient satisfaction.

REFERENCES

Allaouchiche, B., F. Duflo, R. Debon, A. Bergeret, and D. Chassard. 2002. "Noise in the Postanaesthesia Care Unit." *British Journal of Anaesthesia* 88 (3): 369–73.

Bayo, M. V., A. M. Garcia, and A. Garcia. 1995. "Noise Levels in an Urban Hospital and Workers' Subjective Responses." *Archives of Environmental Health* 50 (3): 247–51.

Beauchemin, K. M., and P. Hays. 1996. "Sunny Hospital Rooms Expedite Recovery from Severe and Refractory Depressions." *Journal of Affective Disorders* 40 (1–2): 49–51.

———. 1998. "Dying in the Dark: Sunshine, Gender and Outcomes in Myocardial Infarction." *Journal of the Royal Society of Medicine* 91 (2): 352–54.

Benedetti, F., C. Colombo, B. Barbini, E. Campori, and E. Smeraldi. 2001. "Morning Sunlight Reduces Length of Hospitalization in Bipolar Depression." *Journal of Affective Disorder* 62 (3): 221–23.

Berg, S. 2001. "Impact of Reduced Reverberation Time on Sound-Induced Arousals During Sleep." *Sleep* 24 (3): 289–92.

Berglund, B., T. Lindvall, and D. H. Schwela (eds.). 1999. *Guidelines for Community Noise.* Geneva, Switzerland: World Health Organization.

Blomkvist, V., C. A. Eriksen, T. Theorell, R. Ulrich, and G. Rasmanis. 2005. "Acoustics and Psychosocial Environment in Intensive Coronary Care." *Occupational and Environmental Medicine* 62 (3): e1.

Brandon, D. H., D. Holditch-Davis, and M. Belyea. 2002. "Preterm Infants Born at Less than 3 Weeks' Gestation have Improved Growth in Cycled Light Compared with Continuous Near Darkness." *Journal of Pediatrics* 140 (2): 192–99.

Butler, D., A. L. Acquino, A. A. Hissong, and P. A. Scott. 1993. "Wayfinding by Newcomers in a Complex Building." *Human Factors* 25 (1): 159–73.

Carpman, J., and M. Grant. 1993. *Design that Cares: Planning Health Facilities for Patients and Visitors, 2nd Edition.* Chicago: American Hospital Publishing.

Carpman, J., M. A. Grant, and D. Simmons. 1983–84. "Wayfinding in the Hospital Environment: The Impact of Various Floor Numbering Alternatives." *Journal of Environmental Systems* 13 (4): 353–64.

———. 1984. *No More Mazes: Research about Design for Wayfinding in Hospitals.* Ann Arbor, MI: The University of Michigan Hospitals.

———. 1985. "Hospital Design and Wayfinding: A Video Simulation Study." *Environment & Behavior* 17 (3): 296–314.

Chaudhury, H., A. Mahmood, and M. Valente. 2003. "Pilot Study on Comparative Assessment of Patient Care Issues in Single and Multiple Occupancy Rooms." Unpublished report of the Coalition for Health Environments Research, San Francisco.

Christensen, K. E. 1979. "An Impact Analysis Framework for Calculating the Costs of Staff Disorientation in Hospitals. Wayfinding in Hospital Environments: A School of Architecture and Planning Report Series." University of California School of Architecture and Urban Planning, Los Angeles.

Cohen, S., A. J. Tyrrell, and A. P. Smith. 1991. "Psychological Stress and Susceptibility to the Common Cold." *New England Journal of Medicine* 325 (9): 606–12.

Cooper-Marcus C., and M. Barnes. 1995. *Gardens in Healthcare Facilities: Uses, Therapeutic Benefits, and Design Recommendations*. Concord, CA: The Center for Health Design.

Diette, G. B., N. Lechtzin, E. Haponik, A. Devrotes, and H. R. Rubin. 2003. "Distraction Therapy with Nature Sights and Sounds Reduces Pain During Flexible Bronchoscopy: A Complementary Approach to Routine Analgesia." *Chest* 123 (3): 941–48.

Frumpkin, H. 2001. "Beyond Toxicity: Human Health and the Natural Environment." *American Journal of Preventive Medicine* 20 (3): 234–40.

Gast, P. L., and C. F. Baker. 1989. "The CCU Patient: Anxiety and Annoyance to Noise." *Critical Care Nursing Quarterly* 12 (3): 39–54.

Gatchel, R. J., A. Baum, and D. S. Krantz. 1989. *An Introduction to Health Psychology, 2nd Edition*. New York: McGraw-Hill.

Grover, P. 1971. "Wayfinding in Hospital Environments: UCLA Hospital Disorientation Pilot Case Study." University of California Graduate School of Architecture and Urban Planning, Los Angeles.

Hagerman, I., G. Rasmanis, V. Blomkvist, R. Ulrich, C. A. Eriksen, and T. Theorell. 2005. "Influence of Intensive Coronary Care Acoustics on the Quality of Care and Physiological State of Patients." *International Journal of Cardiology* 98 (2): 267–70.

Haq, S., and C. Zimring. 2003. "Just Down the Road a Piece: The Development of Topological Knowledge of Building Layouts." *Environment & Behavior* 35 (1): 132–60.

Harris, D. 2000. "Environmental Quality and Healing Environments: A Study of Flooring Materials in a Healthcare Telemetry Unit." Ph.D. dissertation, Texas A&M University, College Station, Texas.

Heerwagen, J. 1990. "The Psychological Aspects of Windows and Window Design." In *Proceedings of the 21st Annual Conference of the Environmental Design Research Association,* edited by K. H. Anthony, J. Choi, and B. Orland. Edmond, OK: Environmental Design Research Association.

Hilton, B. A. 1985. "Noise in Acute Patient Care Areas." *Research in Nursing & Health* 8 (3): 283–91.

Hoffman, H. G., J. N. Doctor, D. R. Patterson, G. J. Carrougher, and T. A. Furness, III. 2000. "Virtual Reality as an Adjunctive Pain Control During Burn Wound Care in Adolescent Patients." *Pain* 85(1–2): 305–09.

Holahan, C. J. 1972. "Seating Patterns and Patient Behavior in an Experimental Dayroom." *Journal of Abnormal Psychology* 80 (2): 115–24.

Kaplan, R. 1993. "The Role of Nature in the Context of the Workplace." *Landscape and Urban Planning* 26 (1–4): 193–201.

Kiecolt-Glaser, J. K., R. Glaser, C. Dyer, E. C. Shuttleworth, P. Orgrocki, and C. E. Speicher. 1987. "Chronic Stress and Immune Function in Family Caregivers of Alzheimer's Disease Victims." *Psychosomatic Medicine* 49 (5): 523–35.

Kiecolt-Glaser, J. K., P. T. Marucha, W. B. Malarkey, A. M. Mercado, and R. Glaser. 1995. "Slowing of Wound Healing by Psychological Stress." *Lancet* 346 (8984): 1194–96.

Leather, P., M. Pyrgas, D. Beale, and C. Lawrence. 1998. "Windows in the Workplace: Sunlight, View, and Occupational Stress." *Environment & Behavior* 30 (6): 739–62.

Levine, M., I. Marchon, and G. Hanley. 1984. "The Placement and Misplacement of You-Are-Here Maps." *Environment & Behavior* 16 (2): 139–57.

Lewy, A. J., V. K. Bauer, N. L. Cutler, R. L. Sack, S. Ahmed, K. H. Thomas, M. L. Blood, and J. M. Jackson. 1998. "Morning vs. Evening Light Treatment of Patients with Winter Depression." *Archives of General Psychiatry* 55 (10): 890–96.

Lovell, B. B., S. Ancoli-Israel, and R. Gevirtz. 1995. "Effect of Bright Light Treatment on Agitated Behavior in Institutionalized Elderly Subjects." *Psychiatry Research* 57 (1): 7–12.

McCaul, K. D., and J. M. Malott. 1984. "Distraction and Coping with Pain." *Psychological Bulletin* 95 (3): 516–33.

Melin, L., and K. G. Gotestam. 1981. "The Effects of Rearranging Ward Routines on Communication and Eating Behaviors of Psychogeriatric Patients." *Journal of Applied Behavior Analysis* 14 (1): 47–51.

Melzack, R., and P. D. Wall. 1965. "Pain Mechanisms: A New Theory." *Science* 150 (699): 971–79.

Meyer, T. J., S. E. Eveloff, M. S. Bauer, W. A. Schwartz, N. S. Hill, and R. P. Millman. 1994. "Adverse Environmental Conditions in the Respiratory and Medical ICU Settings." *Chest* 105 (4): 1211–16.

Miller, A. C., L. C. Hickman, and G. K. Lemasters. 1992. "A Distraction Technique for Control of Burn Pain." *Journal of Burn Care and Rehabilitation* 13 (5): 576–80.

Nelson-Shulman, Y. 1983–84. "Information and Environmental Stress: Report of a Hospital Intervention." *Journal of Environmental Systems* 13 (4): 303–16.

Ortega-Andeane, P., and J. Urbina-Soria. 1988. "A Case Study of Wayfinding and Security in a Mexico City Hospital." Paper presented at the Environmental Design Research Association Conference. Pomona, California, May 11–15.

Parthasarathy, S., and M. Tobin. 2004. "Sleep in the Intensive Care Unit." *Intensive Care Medicine* 30 (2): 197–206.

Parsons, R., and T. Hartig. 2000. "Environmental Psychophysiology." In *Handbook of Psychophysiology, 2nd Edition*, edited by J. T. Cacioppo and L. G. Tassinary, 815–46. New York: Cambridge University Press.

Peponis, J., C. Zimring, and Y. K. Choi. 1990. "Finding the Building in Wayfinding." *Environment & Behavior* 22 (5): 555–90.

Press Ganey, Inc. 2003. *National Patient Satisfaction Data for 2003.* South Bend, IN: Press Ganey.

Robertson, A., C. Cooper-Peel, and P. Vos. 1998. "Peak Noise Distribution in the Neonatal Intensive Care Nursery." *Journal of Perinatology* 18 (5): 361–64.

Sallstrom, C., P. O. Sandman, and A. Norberg. 1987. "Relatives' Experience of the Terminal Care of Longterm Geriatric Patients in Open-Plan Rooms." *Scandinavian Journal of Caring Science* 1 (4): 133–40.

Schneider, L. F., and H. A. Taylor. 1999. "How Do You Get There from Here? Mental Representations of Route Descriptions." *Applied Cognitive Psychology* 13 (5): 415–41.

Schneider, S. M., M. Prince-Paul, M. J. Allen, P. Silverman, and D. Talaba. 2004. "Virtual Reality as a Distraction Intervention for Women Receiving Chemotherapy." *Oncology Nursing Forum* 31 (1): 81–88.

Shepley, M. M. 2004. "Evidence-based Design for Infants and Staff in the Neonatal Intensive Care Unit." *Clinical Perinatology* 31 (2): 299–311.

Sherman, S. A., J. W. Varni, R. S. Ulrich, and V. L. Malcarne. Forthcoming. "Post-Occupancy Evaluation of Healing Gardens in a Pediatric Cancer Center." *Landscape and Urban Planning.*

Slevin, M., N. Farrington, G. Duffy, L. Daly, and J. F. Murphy. 2000. "Altering the NICU and Measuring Infants' Responses." *Acta Paediatrica* 89 (5): 577–81.

Southwell, M. T., and G. Wistow. 1995. "Sleep in Hospitals at Night: Are Patients' Needs Being Met?" *Journal of Advanced Nursing* 21 (6): 1101–109.

Terman, J. S., M. Terman, E.-S. Lo, and T. B. Cooper. 2001. "Circadian Time of Morning Light Administration and Therapeutic Response in Winter Depression." *Archives of General Psychiatry* 58 (1): 69–75.

Topf, M., and E. Dillon. 1988. "Noise-Induced Stress as a Predictor of Burnout in Critical Care Nurses." *Heart Lung* 17 (5): 567–74.

Topf, M., and J. Davis. 1993. "Critical Care Unit Noise and Rapid Eye Movement (REM) Sleep." *Heart Lung* 17 (5): 567–74.

Tse, M. M. Y., J. K. F. Ng, J. W. Y. Chung, and T. K. S. Wong. 2002. "The Effect of Visual Stimuli on Pain Threshold and Tolerance." *Journal of Clinical Nursing* 11 (4): 462–69.

Uchino, B. N., and T. S. Garvey. 1997. "The Availability of Social Support Reduces Cardiovascular Reactivity to Acute Psychological Stress." *Journal of Behavioral Medicine* 20 (1): 15–27.

Ulrich R., C. Zimring, W. Quan, and A. Joseph. 2004. "The Role of the Physical Environment in the Hospital of the 21st Century." Concord, CA: The Center for Health Design.

Ulrich, R. S. 1984. "View Through a Window May Influence Recovery from Surgery." *Science* 224 (4647): 420–21.

———. 1991. "Effects of Interior Design on Wellness: Theory and Recent Scientific Research." *Journal of Health Care Interior Design* 3 (1): 97–109.

———. 1999. "Effects of Gardens on Health Outcomes: Theory and Research." In *Healing Gardens*, edited by C. Cooper Marcus and M. Barnes, 27–86. New York: John Wiley & Sons.

Ulrich, R. S., and L. Gilpin. 2003. "Healing Arts: Nutrition for the Soul." In *Putting Patients First: Designing and Practicing Patient-Centered Care*, edited by S. B. Frampton, L. Gilpin, and P. Charmel, 117–46. San Francisco: Jossey-Bass.

Ulrich, R. S., B. Lawson, and M. Martinez. 2003. *Exploring the Patient Environment: An NHS Estates Workshop*. London: The Stationery Office.

Ulrich, R. S., O. Lundén, and J. L. Eltinge. 1993. "Effects of Exposure to Nature and Abstract Pictures on Patients Recovering from Heart Surgery." Paper presented at the 33rd meeting of the Society for Psychophysiological Research. Abstract in *Psychophysiology* 30 (Suppl. 1): 7.

Ulrich, R. S., R. F. Simons, and M. A. Miles. 2003. "Effects of Environmental Simulations and Television on Blood Donor Stress." *Journal of Architectural & Planning Research* 20 (1): 38–47.

Van den Berg, A., S. L. Koole, and N. Y. Van der Wulp. 2003. "Environmental Preference and Restoration: How Are They Related?" *Journal of Environmental Psychology* 23 (2): 135–46.

Van der Ploeg, H. M. 1988. "Stressful Medical Events: A Survey of Patients' Perceptions." In *Topics in Health Psychology*, edited by S. Maies, C. D. Spielberger, P. B. Defares, and I. G. Sarason, 193–203. New York: John Wiley & Sons.

Verderber, S. 1986. "Dimensions of Person-Window Transactions in the Hospital Environment." *Environment & Behavior* 18 (4): 450–66.

Volicer, B. J., M. A. Isenberg, and M. W. Burns. 1977. "Medical-Surgical Differences in Hospital Stress Factors." *Journal of Human Stress* 3 (2): 3–13.

Walch, J. M., B. S. Rabin, R. Day, J. N. Williams, K. Choi, and J. D. Kang. 2005. "The Effect of Sunlight on Post-Operative Analgesic Medication Use: A Prospective Study of Patients Undergoing Spinal Surgery." *Psychosomatic Medicine* 67 (1): 156–63.

Walder, B., D. Francioli, J. J. Meyer, M. Lancon, and J. A. Romand. 2000. "Effects of Guidelines Implementation in a Surgical Intensive Care Unit to Control Nighttime Light and Noise Levels." *Critical Care Medicine* 28 (7): 2242–47.

Whall, A. L., M. E. Black, C. J. Groh, D. J. Yankou, B. J. Kupferschmid, and N. L. Foster. 1997. "The Effect of Natural Environments upon Agitation and Aggression in Late Stage Dementia Patients." *American Journal of Alzheimer's Disease and Other Dementias* (Sept.–Oct.): 216–20.

Whitehouse, S., J. W. Varni, M. Seid, C. Cooper-Marcus, M. J. Ensberg, J. R. Jacobs, et al. 2001. "Evaluating a Children's Hospital Garden Environment: Utilization and Consumer Satisfaction." *Journal of Environmental Psychology* 21 (3): 301–14.

Wright, P., A. J. Hull, and A. Lickorish. 1993. "Navigating in a Hospital Outpatients' Department: The Merits of Maps and Wall Signs." *Journal of Architectural and Planning Research* 10 (1): 76–89.

Yinnon, A. M., Y. Ilan, B. Tadmor, G. Altarescu, and C. Hershko. 1992. "Quality of Sleep in the Medical Department." *British Journal of Clinical Practitioners* 46 (2): 88–91.

Zahr, L. K., and J. de Traversay. 1995. "Premature Infant Responses to Noise Reduction by Earmuffs: Effects on Behavioral and Physiologic Measures." *Journal of Perinatology* 15 (6): 448–55.

Zimring, C. 1990. "The Costs of Confusion: Non-Monetary and Monetary Costs of the Emory University Hospital Wayfinding System." Atlanta: Georgia Institute of Technology.

CHAPTER 4

The Environment's Impact on Safety

Craig Zimring, Ph.D.; Roger Ulrich, Ph.D.; Anjali Joseph; and Xiaobo Quan

U.S. HOSPITALS ARE dangerous and stressful for patients, families, and staff members. Medical errors and hospital-acquired infections are among the leading causes of death in the United States, each killing more Americans than AIDS, breast cancer, or automobile accidents (Institute of Medicine [IOM] 2001). According to IOM's landmark *Crossing the Quality Chasm* report, "The frustration levels of both patients and clinicians have probably never been higher. Yet the problems remain. Health care today harms too frequently and routinely fails to deliver its potential benefits." Problems with U.S. healthcare not only influence patients; they affect staff as well. Registered nurses have a turnover rate averaging 20 percent (Joint Commission on Accreditation of Healthcare Organizations [JCAHO] 2002).

As with Chapter 3, in this chapter we report on some of the results of a large literature review conducted for The Center for Health Design (The Center) in 2004. A large and growing body of rigorous, scientifically defensible research shows that design of the hospital environment affects the safety of patients and staff. Design has a particular role in reducing: (1) airborne and contact-spread hospital-acquired infections, (2) patient falls, and (3) staff errors.

HOSPITAL-ACQUIRED INFECTIONS

Hospital-acquired, or nosocomial, infections pose a serious threat to the health of patients, staff, and visitors in hospitals. According to one study, up to 2 million U.S. hospital patients contract dangerous infections every year during their hospital stays (Weinstein 1998). In 1995 nosocomial infections cost $4.5 billion and contributed to more than 88,000 deaths (Weinstein 1998).

A strong body of research evidence shows that the built environment influences the incidence of infection in hospitals. Person-to-person spread of infections in the healthcare setting can occur via direct contact, droplet, airborne, fecal-oral, and bloodborne routes. The research literature shows that the design of the physical environment influences hospital-acquired infection rates by affecting both airborne and contact transmission routes. The literature suggests a clear pattern in which infection rates are lower with good air quality and single- rather than multi-bed rooms. Also, there is some evidence that providing numerous, easily accessible alcohol-based hand-rub dispensers or sinks can increase hand-washing compliance and thereby reduce contact contamination.

Reducing Airborne Transmission of Infection

Well-conducted research has linked all of the following to air quality and infection rates (Humphreys et al. 1991; Iwen et al. 1994; Loo et al. 1996; Opal et al. 1986; Oren et al. 2001):

- Type of air filter
- Direction of airflow and air pressure
- Air changes per hour in room
- Humidity
- Ventilation system cleaning and maintenance
- Dust or particulate generation during hospital construction and renovation activities

There is convincing evidence that immunocompromised and other high-acuity patient groups have lower incidence of infection when housed in an isolation room with a high-efficiency particulate air (HEPA) filtration system (Passweg et al. 1998; Sherertz and Sullivan 1985; Sherertz et al. 1987). In one study bone marrow transplant recipients assigned to beds outside a HEPA-filtered environment had a tenfold greater incidence of nosocomial Aspergillus infection compared to other immunocompromised patient populations who were in HEPA-filtered spaces (Sherertz et al. 1987).

Air contamination is lowest in laminar airflow rooms with HEPA filters, and this approach is recommended for operating room suites and areas with ultraclean room requirements such as those housing immunocompromised patient populations (Alberti et al. 2001; Arlet et al. 1989; Dharan and Pittet 2002; Friberg, Ardnor, and Lundholm 2003; Hahn et al. 2002; Sherertz et al. 1987).[1] HEPA filters are suggested for healthcare facilities by The Centers for Disease Control and the Healthcare Infection Control Practices Advisory Committee but are either required or strongly recommended in all construction and renovation areas (Sehulster and Chinn 2003).

Effective prevention or control measures during construction and renovation activities include, for example, portable HEPA filters, barriers between the patient care and construction areas, negative air pressure in the construction or renovation area relative to patient care spaces, and sealed patient windows. There is strong evidence of the impact of using HEPA filters for air intakes near construction and renovation sites (Loo et al. 1996; Mahieu et al. 2000; Opal et al. 1986; Oren et al. 2001). Humphreys et al. (1991) demonstrated that HEPA filters are not by themselves an adequate control measure and must be employed in conjunction with other measures such as enhanced cleaning, sealing of windows, and barriers.

Reducing Contact Transmission of Infection

Although infection caused by airborne transmission poses a major safety problem, most infections are now acquired in the hospital via the contact pathway (Bauer et al. 1990; IOM 2004). Many environmental surfaces and features become contaminated near infected patients. Examples of surfaces found to be contaminated frequently via contact with patients and staff include overbed tables, bed privacy curtains, computer keyboards, infusion pump buttons, door handles, bedside rails, blood pressure cuffs, chairs and other furniture, and countertops (Aygun et al. 2002; Boyce et al. 1997; Bures et al. 2000; Devine, Cooke, and Wright 2001; Neely and Maley 2001; Noskin et al. 2000; Palmer 1999; Roberts, Findlay, and Lang 2001; Rountree et al. 1967; Sanderson and Weissler 1992; Williams, Singh, and Romberg 2003). These and other contaminated surfaces act as pathogen reservoirs that increase cross-infection risk. Boyce et al. (1997) found that in the rooms of patients infected with methicillin-resistant Staphylococcus aureus (MRSA) 27 percent of all environmental surfaces sampled were contaminated with MRSA.

Reducing Infections by Increased Hand Washing

It is well-established that the hands of healthcare staff are the principal cause of contact transmission of pathogens from patient to patient (Larson 1988). Accordingly, the importance of assiduous hand washing by healthcare workers cannot be overemphasized for reducing hospital-acquired infections. In this context the fact that rates of hand washing by healthcare staff are low represents a serious patient safety challenge. Several studies of hand washing in high-acuity units with vulnerable patients have found that as few as one in seven staff members washes their hands between patients. Compliance rates in the range of 15 percent to 35 percent are typical; rates above 40 percent to 50 percent are the exception (Albert and Condie 1981; Graham 1990). Hand-washing compliance tends to be consistently lower in units that are understaffed and have a high patient census or bed occupancy rate (Archibald et al. 1997).

Educational programs to increase hand-washing adherence have yielded disappointing, or at best mixed, results. Some investigations have found that educational interventions generate no increase at all in hand washing. Even intensive education or training programs (e.g., classes, group feedback) produce only transient increases in hand washing (Conly et al. 1989; Dorsey, Cydulka, and Emerman 1996; Dubbert et al. 1990). Given the tremendous morbidity and mortality associated with high rates of hospital-acquired infections, there is an urgent need to identify more effective ways for producing sustained increases in hand washing.

At least six studies have examined whether hand washing is improved by increasing the ratio of the number of sinks or hand-cleaner dispensers to beds or by placing sinks or hand-cleaner dispensers in more accessible locations (Cohen et al. 2003; Graham 1990; Kaplan and McGuckin 1986; Muto, Sistrom, and Farr 2000; Pittet et al. 2000; Vernon et al. 2003). These studies offer support, albeit limited, for the notion that providing numerous, conveniently located alcohol-rub dispensers or washing sinks can increase compliance.

In particular, the evidence suggests that installing alcohol-based hand-cleaner dispensers at bedsides usually improves adherence. For example, Pittet et al. (2000) found that a combination of bedside antiseptic hand-rub dispensers and posters to remind staff to clean their hands substantially increased compliance. By contrast, Muto, Sistrom, and Farr (2000) reported that placing alcohol-gel dispensers next to the doors of patient rooms did not increase adherence. Two other investigations focusing on sinks (water and soap) identified a positive relationship between observed frequency of hand washing and a higher ratio of sinks to beds (Kaplan and McGuckin 1986; Vernon et al. 2003). Providing automated water-and-soap sinks, however, appears not to increase hand-washing rates compared to traditional nonautomated sinks (Larson et al. 1991, 1997).

Furthermore, three studies offer convincing and important evidence that providing each single-patient room with a conveniently located sink reduces nosocomial infection rates in intensive care units (ICUs), such as neonatal intensive care or burn units, compared to when the same staff and comparable patients are in multibed open units with few sinks (Goldmann, Durbin, and Freeman 1981; McManus et al. 1985, 1994; Mulin et al. 1997). Although hand-washing frequency was not measured in these studies, the investigators posited that increased hand washing was an important factor in reducing infections in the units with single rooms and more sinks.

A comparison of an ICU converted from an open unit with few sinks to single rooms with one sink per room found a tendency for hand washing to increase (from 16 percent to 30 percent) but no decline in infection incidence (Preston, Larson, and Stamm 1981). These results are perhaps explainable by the fact that several sinks in the single-bed unit were placed in comparatively inaccessible or inconvenient locations such as behind doors or away from staff work paths.

Reducing Infections with Single-Bed Rooms

We also identified at least 16 studies relevant to the question of whether nosocomial infection rates differ between single- and multi-bed rooms. Together, the findings provide a strong pattern of evidence indicating that infection rates are usually lower in single-bed rooms. Different mechanisms or factors have been implicated as contributing to lower infection incidence in single rooms, including lower patient-to-patient airborne infection and reduced contact infection as a result of easier cleaning.

One clear set of advantages relates to reducing airborne transmission through air quality and ventilation measures such as HEPA filters, negative room pressure to prevent a patient with an aerial-spread infection from infecting others, or maintaining positive pressure to protect an immunocompromised patient from airborne pathogens in nearby rooms.

Passweg et al. (1998) found that the combination of room isolation and HEPA filtration reduced infection and mortality in bone marrow transplant patients and significantly increased their one-year survival rates. Research studying burn patients also has shown that single rooms and good air quality substantially reduce infection incidence and mortality (McManus et al. 1992, 1994; Shirani et al. 1986; Thompson, Meredith, and Molnar 2002). Studies of cross-infection for contagious airborne diseases (e.g., influenza, measles, tuberculosis) have found, as would be expected, that placing patients in single rooms is safer than housing them in multi-bed spaces (Gardner et al. 1973; McKendrick and Emond 1976).

Severe acute respiratory syndrome (SARS) outbreaks in Asia and Canada dramatically highlighted the shortcomings of multi-bed rooms for controlling or preventing infections both for patients and healthcare workers. SARS is transmitted by droplets that can be airborne over limited areas. Approximately 75 percent of SARS cases in Toronto resulted from exposure in hospital settings (Farquharson and Baguley 2003). The pervasiveness of multi-bed spaces in Canadian and Asian emergency departments and ICUs, together with the scarcity of isolation rooms with negative pressure, severely hindered treatment and control measures. Toronto hospitals were forced to create additional negative-pressure isolation rooms by quickly constructing wall barriers to replace bed curtains and making airflow and pressure adaptations (Farquharson and Baguley 2003).

In addition to clear advantages in reducing airborne transmission, several studies show that single-bed rooms lessen the risk of infections acquired by contact. As mentioned earlier, many surfaces in patient rooms become reservoirs for pathogens through contact with patients and staff. Compared to single-bed rooms, multi-bed rooms are far more difficult to decontaminate thoroughly after a patient is discharged and therefore worsen the problem of multiple surfaces acting as pathogen reservoirs. Because different staff members who enter a room can touch the same contaminated surfaces, the risk of a nurse unknowingly becoming contaminated should be greater in multi-bed rooms.

Circumstantial support for this point is provided by research on contamination of nurses in units housing MRSA-infected patients. Boyce et al. (1997) found that 42 percent of nurses who had no direct contact with an MRSA patient but had touched contaminated surfaces contaminated their gloves with MRSA.

PATIENT FALLS

An extensive literature looks at the causes and risk factors involved in patient falls in hospitals. This is an area of great importance because patients who fall incur physical injuries, psychological effects, and longer lengths of stay in the hospital (Brandis 1999). It is estimated that the total cost of fall injuries for older people was around $20.2 billion per year in the United States in 1994; this figure is projected to reach $32.4 billion (in 1994 U.S. dollars) in 2020 (Chang et al. 2004).

Although the role of the environment in causing or preventing patient falls is widely accepted, there is not yet conclusive evidence correlating environmental interventions with reduced falls. Available studies usually examine the location of fall incidents retrospectively or discuss environmental modification programs such as improving lighting and securing carpeting. However, a meta-analysis and systematic review of randomized controlled trials of fall-prevention interventions found no clear evidence for the independent effectiveness of environmental modification programs (Chang et al. 2004).

Nevertheless, several studies have shown that most patient falls occur in the bedroom, followed by the bathroom, and that comprehensive fall-prevention programs can have an effect. Brandis (1999) reported transfers to and from bed as the cause of approximately 42 percent of inpatient falls. Design faults identified in the bathroom and bedroom areas included slippery floors, inappropriate door openings, poor placement of rails and accessories, and incorrect toilet and furniture heights. After the fall-prevention program (which included identifying high-risk patients, management strategies, environmental and equipment modification, and standardization) was implemented, falls decreased by approximately 17 percent. Thus, fall-prevention strategies that have included environmental modification have worked in the past. However, it is not clear how much of the effectiveness of such strategies can be attributed to environmental factors alone.

An innovative and promising environmental strategy for reducing falls has its origins in evidence suggesting that many falls occur when patients attempt to get out of bed unassisted or unobserved (Uden 1985; Vassallo et al. 2000). It should be mentioned that there is considerable evidence that bedrails are not effective for reducing the incidence of falls and may actually increase the severity of fall injuries from beds (Capezuti et al. 2002; Hanger, Ball, and Wood 1999; van Leeuwen et al. 2001).

To increase observation and improve assistance for patients and thereby reduce falls, Methodist Hospital in Indianapolis, Indiana, changed its coronary critical care unit with a centralized nurses' station and two-bed rooms to one with decentralized nurses' stations and large single-bed rooms designed to support family presence (Hendrich, Fay, and Sorrells 2002). Comparison of data from two years prior to and three years after the unit redesign showed that falls were cut by two-thirds—from six to two per 1,000 patients. Given that falls are a critical safety problem, additional research is needed to understand the effectiveness of this approach for designing patient care units.

INCREASED STAFF EFFECTIVENESS AND REDUCED ERRORS

The jobs of nurses, physicians, and others often require a complex choreography of direct patient care, critical communications, charting, filling prescriptions, accessing technology and information, and other tasks. Many hospital settings have not been rethought as jobs have changed; as a result, the design of hospitals often increases staff stress and reduces their effectiveness in delivering care. Although much research in the hospital setting has been aimed at patients, a growing and compelling body of evidence suggests that improved designs can make the jobs of staff much easier.

Workplace design that reflects a closer alignment of work patterns and the physical setting, such as redesign of a pharmacy layout, has been shown to improve workflow and reduce waiting times as well as increase patient satisfaction with the service (Pierce et al. 1990). Other studies that compared delivery times in decentralized and centralized pharmacy systems found medication delivery times were reduced by more than 50 percent by using decentralized drug-dose distribution systems (Hibbard et al. 1981; Reynolds, Johnson, and Longe 1978).

Reducing Medication Errors

The IOM report on the high prevalence of medical errors has encouraged a more careful look at the sources of error in healthcare. Much of this work has been influenced by the seminal work of James Reason (2000). Reason argues that most errors are best seen as the result of a defective system rather than of careless individuals and that in fact most individuals are doing the best they can. A robust and effective system is one that increases patient safety by reducing active errors—those of commission, such as prescribing or administering the wrong medication—by creating latent conditions that do not overtax individuals' abilities to make careful decisions, and through reasoned systems. An effective system also establishes multiple checks that catch errors, which are inevitable in any complex system, and recovers from them before they have negative consequences.

These concepts are well-supported by the research literature. For example, dispensing error rates by hospital pharmacists decline steeply when interruptions or distractions, such as telephone calls or remarks from other staff, are reduced or eliminated (Flynn et al. 1999). This suggests that spaces or rooms for dispensing medications should be separate and isolated from the distractions and interruptions of nursing stations.

Other studies have found that medication error rates also can be lowered by providing appropriate—usually brighter—work illumination levels. A large-scale controlled study of hospital pharmacists found that medication dispensing errors occurred more frequently when work surface illumination levels were in the low to moderate range (450 to 1,000 lux) (Buchanan et al. 1991). The same pharmacists made substantially fewer errors, however, when work surface illumination levels were increased to 1,500 lux.

The finding that bright lighting reduces medication errors suggests that the lowered illumination levels (200 to 500 lux) found in many healthcare spaces, because of greater use of computer terminals and pressures to reduce electricity costs, may be too low. Much research has shown that people over the age of 40 require higher illumination for reading and other visual tasks, and the average age of a nurse in the United States is 47. The aging of the nursing work force in the United States and elsewhere therefore implies that work-surface illumination levels of 1,500 to 2,000 lux may be needed to lessen medication errors when performing paper-based reading and writing tasks.

There is increasing evidence that medical errors, including medication errors, can be markedly lowered by reducing the transfer of patients between rooms or different types of units (Cook, Render, and Woods 2000; Hendrich, Fay, and Sorrells 2004; IOM 2004). When patients are transferred, many things can go wrong and often do. Reasons that transfers produce errors and worsen safety include, for instance, changes in staff caring for a patient, communication discontinuities, loss of information, changes in systems and computers, and delays or interruptions in patients receiving medications and care. Multi-bed rooms have been shown to generate many more transfers than single-bed rooms because of incompatibility among roommates.

If transfers generate errors, it follows that errors should be reduced if the care process and physical patient environment are reorganized and redesigned to eliminate most transfers. One proven approach for achieving this involves an acuity-adaptable care process and staffing model in combination with large single-bed patient rooms equipped with gas outlets and other equipment permitting the room to flex up or down in acuity according to the condition of the patient. When Methodist Hospital changed to acuity-adaptable single-bed rooms in its coronary ICU, transfers declined by 90 percent and medication errors were correspondingly lowered by 70 percent (Hendrich, Fay, and Sorrells 2004).

CONCLUSION

A strong and growing body of scientific evidence shows that the design of hospitals affects patient safety. Effective filtering of the air and special vigilance during construction can reduce airborne infection, and providing single-patient rooms can significantly reduce contact infection. Providing frequent hand-washing stations or alcohol rubs can increase hand washing by staff and reduce infections. Single rooms along with careful preventive programs can reduce patient falls. Improved hospital design can reduce errors by replacing chaotic, stressful conditions with quieter, better lit, more supportive settings that allow careful decision making and multiple checks for error.

NOTE

1. Laminar flows are even, smooth, low-velocity airflows used in clean rooms and other settings where high-quality ventilation is critical. But laminar flows are relatively expensive and difficult to achieve because furnishings, vents, and other features can create turbulence. Cornet et al. (1999) concluded that carefully directed airflow (i.e., laminar airflow) is important. However, we were unable to find and document cost-benefit analysis in the literature to justify the expense versus effectiveness of laminar airflow for patient care areas near construction and renovation sites.

REFERENCES

Albert, R. K., and F. Condie. 1981. "Hand-Washing Patterns in Medical Intensive-care Units." *New England Journal of Medicine* 304 (24): 1465–66.

Alberti, C., A. Bouakline, P. Ribaud, C. Lacroix, P. Rousselot, T. Leblanc, and F. Derouin. 2001. "Relationship Between Environmental Fungal Contamination and the Incidence of Invasive Aspergillosis in Haematology Patients." *Journal of Hospital Infection* 48 (3): 198–206.

Archibald, L. K., M. L. Manning, L. M. Bell, S. Banerjee, and W. R. Jarvis. 1997. "Patient Density, Nurse-to-Patient Ratio and Nosocomial Infection Risk in a Pediatric Cardiac Intensive Care Unit." *Pediatric Infectious Disease Journal* 16 (11): 1045–48.

Arlet, G., E. Gluckman, F. Gerber, Y. Perol, and A. Hirsch. 1989. "Measurement of Bacterial and Fungal Air Counts in Two Bone Marrow Transplant Units." *Journal of Hospital Infection* 13 (1): 63–69.

Aygun, G., O. Demirkiran, T. Utku, B. Mete, S. Urkmez, M. Yilmaz, H. Yasar, Y. Dikmen, and R. Ozturk. 2002. "Environmental Contamination During a Carbapenem-Resistant Acinetobacter Baumannii Outbreak in an Intensive Care Unit." *Journal of Hospital Infection* 52 (4): 259–62.

Bauer, T. M., E. Ofner, H. M. Just, H. Just, and F. D. Daschner. 1990. "An Epidemiological Study Assessing the Relative Importance of Airborne and Direct Contact Transmission of Microorganisms in a Medical Intensive Care Unit." *Journal of Hospital Infection* 15 (4): 301–09.

Boyce, J. M., G. Potter-Bynoe, C. Chenevert, and T. King. 1997. "Environmental Contamination Due to Methicilin-Resistant Staphylococcus Aureus: Possible Infection Control Implications." *Infection Control and Hospital Epidemiology* 18 (9): 622–27.

Brandis, S. 1999. "A Collaborative Occupational Therapy and Nursing Approach to Falls Prevention in Hospital Inpatients." *Journal of Quality in Clinical Practice* 19 (4): 215–21.

Buchanan, T. L., K. N. Barker, J. T. Gibson, B. C. Jiang, and R. E. Pearson. 1991. "Illumination and Errors in Dispensing." *American Journal of Hospital Pharmacy* 48 (10): 2137–45.

Bures, S., J. T. Fishbain, C. F. Uyehara, J. M. Parker, and B. W. Berg. 2000. "Computer Keyboards and Faucet Handles as Reservoirs of Nosocomial Pathogens in the Intensive Care Unit." *American Journal of Infection Control* 28 (6): 465–71.

Capezuti, E., G. Maislin, N. Strumpf, and L. K. Evans. 2002. "Side Rail Use and Bed-Related Fall Outcomes Among Nursing Home Residents." *Journal of the American Geriatrics Society* 50 (1): 90–96.

Chang, J. T., S. C. Morton, L. Z. Rubenstein, W. A. Mojica, M. Maglione, M. J. Suttorp, E. A. Roth, and P. G. Shekelle. 2004. "Interventions for the Prevention of Falls in Older Adults: Systematic Review and Meta-Analysis of Randomised Clinical Trials." *British Medical Journal* 328 (7441): 680.

Cohen, B., L. Saiman, J. Cimiotti, and E. Larson. 2003. "Factors Associated with Hand Hygiene Practices in Two Neonatal Intensive Care Units." *Pediatric Infectious Diseases Journal* 22 (6): 494–99.

Conly, J. M., S. Hill, J. Ross, J. Lertzman, and T. J. Louie. 1989. "Handwashing Practices in an Intensive Care Unit: The Effects of an Educational Program and its Relationship to Infection Rates." *American Journal of Infection Control* 17 (6): 330–39.

Cook, R. I., M. Render, and D. D. Woods. 2000. "Gaps in the Continuity of Care and Progress on Patient Safety." *British Medical Journal* 320 (7237): 791–94.

Cornet, M., V. Levy, L. Fleury, J. Lortholary, S. Barquins, M. H. Coureul, E. Deliere, R. Zittoun, G. Bracker, and A. Bouvet. 1999. "Efficacy of Prevention by High-Efficiency Particulate Air Filtration or Laminar Airflow Against Aspergillus Airborne Contamination During Hospital Renovation." *Infection Control and Hospital Epidemiology* 20 (7): 508–13.

Devine, J., R. P. Cooke, and E. P. Wright. 2001. "Is Methicillin-Resistant Staphylococcus Aureus (MRSA) Contamination of Ward-based Computer Terminals a Surrogate Marker for Nosocomial MRSA Transmission and Handwashing Compliance?" *Journal of Hospital Infection* 48 (1): 72–75.

Dharan, S., and D. Pittet. 2002. "Environmental Controls in Operating Theatres." *Journal of Hospital Infection* 51 (2): 79–84.

Dorsey, S. T., R. K. Cydulka, and C. L. Emerman. 1996. "Is Handwashing Teachable? Failure to Improve Handwashing Behavior in an Urban Emergency Department." *Academy of Emergency Medicine* 3 (4): 360–65.

Dubbert, P. M., J. Dolce, W. Richter, M. Miller, and S. W. Chapman. 1990. "Increasing ICU Staff Handwashing: Effects of Education and Group Feedback." *Infection Control and Hospital Epidemiology* 11 (4): 191–93.

Farquharson, C., and K. Baguley. 2003. "Responding to the Severe Acute Respiratory Syndrome (SARS) Outbreak: Lessons Learned in a Toronto Emergency Department." *Journal of Emergency Nursing* 29 (3): 222–28.

Flynn, E. A., K. N. Barker, J. T. Gibson, R. E. Pearson, B. A. Berger, and L. A. Smith. 1999. "Impact of Interruptions and Distractions on Dispensing Errors in an Ambulatory Care Pharmacy." *American Journal of Health Systems Pharmacy* 56 (13): 1319–25.

Friberg, S., B. Ardnor, and R. Lundholm. 2003. "The Addition of a Mobile Ultra-Clean Exponential Laminar Airflow Screen to Conventional Operating Room Ventilation Reduces Bacterial Contamination to Operating Box Levels." *Journal of Hospital Infection* 55 (2): 92–97.

Gardner, P. S., S. D. Court, J. T. Brocklebank, M. A. Downham, and D. Weightman. 1973. "Virus Cross-Infection in Pediatric Wards." *British Medical Journal* 2 (5866): 571–75.

Goldmann, D. A., W. A. Durbin, Jr., and J. Freeman. 1981. "Nosocomial Infections in a Neonatal Intensive Care Unit." *Journal of Infectious Diseases* 144 (5): 449–59.

Graham, M. 1990. "Frequency and Duration of Handwashing in an Intensive Care Unit." *American Journal of Infection Control* 18 (2): 77–81.

Hahn, T., K. M. Cummings, A. M. Michalek, B. J. Lipman, B. H. Segal, and P. L. McCarthy, Jr. 2002. "Efficacy of High-Efficiency Particulate Air Filtration in Preventing Aspergillosis in Immunocompromised Patients with Hematologic Malignancies." *Infection Control and Hospital Epidemiology* 23 (9): 525–31.

Hanger, H. C., M. C. Ball, and L. A. Wood. 1999. "An Analysis of Falls in the Hospital: Can We Do Without Bedrails?" *Journal of the American Geriatrics Society* 47 (5): 529–31.

Hendrich, A., J. Fay, and A. Sorrells. 2002. "Courage to Heal: Comprehensive Cardiac Critical Care." *Healthcare Design* (September): 11–13.

———. 2004. "Effects of Acuity-Adaptable Rooms on Flow of Patients and Delivery of Care." *American Journal of Critical Care* 13 (1): 35–45.

Hibbard, F. J., J. A. Bosso, L. W. Sward, and S. Baum. 1981. "Delivery Time in a Decentralized Pharmacy System Without Satellites." *American Journal of Hospital Pharmacy* 38 (5): 690–92.

Humphreys, H., E. M. Johnson, D. W. Warnock, S. M. Willatts, R. J. Winter, and D. C. Speller. 1991. "An Outbreak of Aspergillosis in a General ITU." *Journal of Hospital Infection* 18 (3): 167–77.

Institute of Medicine. 2001. *Crossing the Quality Chasm: A New Health System for the 21st Century.* Washington, DC: National Academies Press.

———. 2004. *Keeping Patients Safe: Transforming the Work Environment of Nurses.* Washington, DC: National Academies Press.

Iwen, P. C., J. C. Davis, E. C. Reed, B. A. Winfield, and S. H. Hinrichs. 1994. "Airborne Fungal Spore Monitoring in a Protective Environment During Hospital Construction, and Correlation with an Outbreak of Invasive Aspergillosis." *Infection Control and Hospital Epidemiology* 15 (5): 303–06.

Joint Commission on Accreditation of Healthcare Organizations. 2002. *Health Care at the Crossroads: Strategies for Addressing the Evolving Nursing Crisis.* Oakbrook Terrace, IL: JCAHO.

Kaplan, L. M., and M. McGuckin. 1986. "Increasing Handwashing Compliance with More Accessible Sinks." *Infection Control* 7 (8): 408–10.

Larson, E. 1988. "A Causal Link Between Handwashing and Risk of Infection? Examination of the Evidence." *Infection Control* 9 (1): 28–36.

Larson, E. L., J. L. Bryan, L. M. Adler, and C. Blane. 1997. "A Multifaceted Approach to Changing Handwashing Behavior." *American Journal of Infection Control* 25 (1): 3–10.

Larson, E., A. McGeer, Z. A. Quraishi, D. Krenzischek, B. J. Parsons, J. Holdford, and W. J. Hierholzer. 1991. "Effect of an Automated Sink on Handwashing Practices and Attitudes in High-Risk Units." *Infection Control and Hospital Epidemiology* 12 (7): 422–28.

Loo, V. G., C. Bertrand, C. Dixon, D. Vitye, B. DeSalis, A. P. McLean, A. Brox, and H. G. Robson. 1996. "Control of Construction-Associated Nosocomial Aspergillosis in an Antiquated Hematology Unit." *Infection Control and Hospital Epidemiology* 17 (6): 360–64.

Mahieu, L. M., J. J. De Dooy, F. A. Van Laer, H. Jansens, and M. M. Leven. 2000. "A Prospective Study on Factors Influencing Aspergillus Spore Load in the Air During Renovation Works in a Neonatal Intensive Care Unit." *Journal of Hospital Infection* 45 (3): 191–97.

McKendrick, G. D., and R. T. Emond. 1976. "Investigation of Cross-Infection in Isolation Wards of Different Design." *Journal of Hygiene (Lond)* 76 (1): 23–31.

McManus, A. T., A. D. Mason, Jr., W. F. McManus, and B. A. Pruitt, Jr. 1992. "Control of Pseudomonas Aeruginosa Infections in Burned Patients." *Surgical Research Communications* 120 (2): 61–67.

———. 1994. "A Decade of Reduced Gram-Negative Infections and Mortality Associated with Improved Isolation of Burned Patients." *Archives of Surgery* 129 (12): 1306–09.

McManus, A. T., W. F. McManus, A. D. Mason, Jr., A. R. Aitcheson, and B. A. Pruitt, Jr. 1985. "Microbial Colonization in a New Intensive Care Burn Unit. A Prospective Cohort Study." *Archives of Surgery* 120 (2): 217–23.

Mulin, B., C. Rouget, C. Clement, P. Bailly, M. C. Julliot, J. F. Viel, M. Thouverez, I. Vieille, F. Barale, and D. Talon. 1997. "Association of Private Isolation Rooms with Ventilator-Associated Acinetobacter Baumannii Pneumonia in a Surgical Intensive-Care Unit." *Infection Control and Hospital Epidemiology* 18 (7): 499–503.

Muto, C. A., M. G. Sistrom, and B. M. Farr. 2000. "Hand Hygiene Rates Unaffected by Installation of Dispensers of a Rapidly Acting Hand Antiseptic." *American Journal of Infection Control* 28 (3): 273–76.

Neely, A. N., and M. P. Maley. 2001. "Dealing with Contaminated Computer Keyboards and Microbial Survival." *American Journal of Infection Control* 29 (2): 131–32.

Noskin, G. A., P. Bednarz, T. Suriano, A. Reiner, and L. Peterson. 2000. "Persistent Contamination of Fabric-Covered Furniture by Vancomycin-Resistant Enterocci: Implication for Upholstery Selection in Hospitals." *American Journal of Infection Control* 28 (4): 311–13.

Opal, S. M., A. A. Asp, P. B. Cannady, Jr., P. L. Morse, L. J. Burton, and P. G. Hammer, II. 1986. "Efficacy of Infection Control Measures During a Nosocomial Outbreak of Disseminated Aspergillosis Associated with Hospital Construction." *Journal of Infectious Diseases* 153 (3): 634–37.

Oren, I., N. Haddad, R. Finkelstein, and J. M. Rowe. 2001. "Invasive Pulmonary Aspergillosis in Neutropenic Patients During Hospital Construction: Before and After Chemoprophylaxis and Institution of HEPA Filters." *American Journal of Hematology* 66 (4): 257–62.

Palmer, R. 1999. "Bacterial Contamination of Curtains in Clinical Areas." *Nursing Standard* 14 (2): 33–35.

Passweg, J. R., P. A. Rowlings, K. A. Atkinson, A. J. Barrett, R. P. Gale, A. Gratwohl, N. Jacobsen, J. P. Klein, P. Ljungman, J. A. Russell, U. W. Schaefer, K. A. Sobocinski, J. M. Vossen, M. J. Zhang, and M. M. Horowitz. 1998. "Influence of Protective Isolation on Outcome of Allogeneic Bone Marrow Transplantation for Leukemia." *Bone Marrow Transplant* 21 (12): 1231–38.

Pierce, R. A., II, E. M. Rogers, M. H. Sharp, and M. Musulin. 1990. "Outpatient Pharmacy Redesign to Improve Work Flow, Waiting Time, and Patient Satisfaction." *American Journal of Hospital Pharmacy* 47 (2): 351–56.

Pittet, D., S. Hugonnet, S. Harbarth, P. Mourouga, V. Sauvan, S. Touveneau, and T. V. Perneger. 2000. "Effectiveness of a Hospital-Wide Programme to Improve Compliance with Hand Hygiene." *Lancet* 356 (9238): 1307–12.

Preston, G. A., E. L. Larson, and W. E. Stamm. 1981. "The Effect of Private Isolation Rooms on Patient Care Practices, Colonization and Infection an Intensive Care Unit." *American Journal of Medicine* 70 (3): 641–45.

Reason, J. 2000. "Human Error: Models and Management." *British Medical Journal* 320 (7237): 768–70.

Reynolds, D. M., M. H. Johnson, and R. L. Longe. 1978. "Medication Delivery Time Requirements in Centralized and Decentralized Unit Dose Drug Distribution Systems." *American Journal of Hospital Pharmacy* 35 (8): 941–43.

Roberts, S. A., R. Findlay, and S. D. Lang. 2001. "Investigation of an Outbreak of Multi-Drug Resistant Acinetobacter Baumannii in an Intensive Care Burns Unit." *Journal of Hospital Infection* 48 (3): 228–32.

Rountree, P. M., M. A. Beard, J. Loewenthal, J. May, and S. B. Renwick. 1967. "Staphylococcal Sepsis in a New Surgical Ward." *British Medical Journal* 1 (533): 132–37.

Sanderson, P. J., and S. Weissler. 1992. "Recovery of Coliforms from the Hands of Nurses and Patients: Activities Leading to Contamination." *Journal of Hospital Infection* 21 (2): 85–93.

Sehulster, L., and R. Y. Chinn. 2003. "Guidelines for Environmental Infection Control in Health-Care Facilities. Recommendations of CDC and the Healthcare Infection Control Practices Advisory Committee (HICPAC)." *MMWR Recommendation Report* 52 (RR-10): 1–42.

Sherertz, R., A. J. Belani, B. S. Kramer, G. J. Elfenbein, R. S. Weiner, M. L. Sullivan, R. G. Thomas, and G. P. Samsa. 1987. "Impact of Air Filtration on Nosocomial Aspergillus Infections: Unique Risk of Bone Marrow Transplant Recipients." *American Journal of Medicine* 83 (4): 709–18.

Sherertz, R. J., and M. L. Sullivan. 1985. "An Outbreak of Infections with Acinetobacter Calcoaceticus in Burn Patients: Contamination of Patients' Mattresses." *Journal of Infectious Diseases* 151 (2): 252–58.

Shirani, K. Z., A. T. McManus, G. M. Vaughan, W. F. McManus, B. A. Pruitt, Jr., and A. D. Mason, Jr. 1986. "Effects of Environment on Infection in Burn Patients." *Archives of Surgery* 121 (1): 31–36.

Thompson, J. T., J. W. Meredith, and J. A. Molnar. 2002. "The Effect of Burn Nursing Units on Burn Wound Infections." *Journal of Burn Care Rehabilitation* 23 (4): 281–86.

Uden, G. 1985. "Inpatient Accidents in Hospitals." *Journal of the American Geriatrics Society* 33 (12): 833–41.

van Leeuwen, M., L. Bennett, S. West, V. Wiles, and J. Grasso. 2001. "Patient Falls from Bed and the Role of Bedrails in the Acute Care Setting." *Australian Journal of Advanced Nursing* 19 (2): 8–13.

Vassallo, M., T. Azeem, M. F. Pirwani, J. C. Sharma, and S. C. Allen. 2000. "An Epidemiological Study of Falls on Integrated General Medical Wards." *International Journal of Clinical Practice* 54 (10): 654–57.

Vernon, M. O., W. E. Trick, S. F. Welbel, B. J. Peterson, and R. A. Weinstein. 2003. "Adherence with Hand Hygiene: Does Number of Sinks Matter?" *Infection Control and Hospital Epidemiology* 24 (3): 224–25.

Weinstein, R. A. 1998. "Nosocomial Infection Update." *Emerging Infectious Diseases* 4 (3): 416–20

Williams, H. N., R. Singh, and E. Romberg. 2003. "Surface Contamination in the Dental Operatory: A Comparison Over Two Decades." *Journal of the American Dental Association* 134 (3): 325–30.

CHAPTER 5

Environmentally Responsible Hospitals

Greg Roberts, AIA, FCSI, ACHA, LEED AP, and
Robin Guenther, AIA, LEED AP

"Sustainable development is the most vibrant and powerful force to impact the building design and construction field in more than a decade" (Cassidy 2003). In every market sector building owners and their architects and constructors are transforming the U.S. construction industry. Fueled by the success of the U.S. Green Building Council's Leadership in Energy and Environmental Design (LEED) rating system, growing federal and state tax credit programs, and public and private financial energy incentives, more than 4.5 percent of construction activity in the United States is seeking to define sustainable building (Lounsbury 2003). The healthcare sector faces unique opportunities and challenges as the construction industry increases its understanding of the impact of the built environment on the health of building occupants, local communities, and global ecosystems.

The healthcare industry has an essential role to play in developing buildings that demonstrate the economic, social, and environmental benefits of green building in the context of high-performance healing environments.

As stated in Chapter 1, the U.S. healthcare system is in the midst of an impressive construction boom. Nationally, the healthcare industry employs 4.5 million workers, accounting for 6 percent of the total commercial workforce. National health expenditures account for more than 13 percent of the gross domestic product, and 31.8 million inpatients were discharged from the nation's hospitals in 1998 (National Center for Health Statistics 1998).

The numbers illustrate that while healthcare provides medical service in the community, the industry is also a significant employer. Likewise, the industry is a major consumer of resources and producer of wastes, accounting for 11 percent of all commercial energy consumption (Energy Information Administration 1996) and diverting 6,600 tons of solid waste to the nation's landfills each day (American Society of Healthcare Environmental Services 1993).

The sheer quantity of construction activity and its effects present a defining opportunity to use sustainable design principles to build better, healthier healthcare buildings that improve patient outcomes, and provide safe and productive work environments for staff while delivering improved financial performance over a typical 40-year existence. Accomplishing these goals challenges the healthcare industry to return to its roots—to "first, do no harm"—and use evidence-based design, materials assessment methodologies, and sustainable building tools to define high-performance healing environments.

Michael Lerner, M.D. (2000), issued this challenge: "The question is whether healthcare professionals can begin to recognize the environmental consequences of our operations and put our own house in order. This is no trivial question." Figure 5.1 illustrates the implied relationship between human health, medical treatment, and environmental pollution that directly affects the mission of the healthcare industry (Bristol Meyers Squibb 2004).

As the healthcare industry's environmental footprint negatively affects the environment, these environmental impacts may in turn affect human health, and human health issues further increase the need for healthcare services. This is the center of the sustainability challenge. Improved environmental performance may contribute to an improved community health status.

Figure 5.1: Interrelationship Between Environmental Pollution and Healthcare

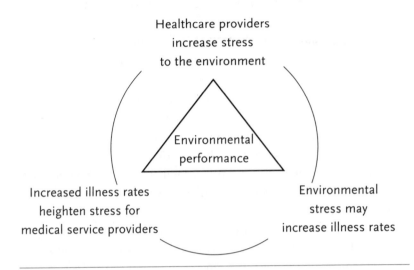

Healthcare providers increase stress to the environment

Environmental performance

Increased illness rates heighten stress for medical service providers

Environmental stress may increase illness rates

THE TRIPLE BOTTOM LINE FOR HEALTH

The fact that the healthcare industry has a responsibility beyond the economic bottom line cannot be denied. David Lawrence (2000) former CEO of Kaiser Permanente, said, "Just as we have responsibility for providing quality patient care [and] . . . keeping our facilities and technology up to date, we have a responsibility for providing leadership in the environment." Lloyd Dean (2000), of Catholic Healthcare West, agreed: "We will not have healthy individuals, healthy families, and healthy communities if we do not have clean air, clean water, and healthy soil." Only by recognizing this bond between humankind and the natural world—and the need for mutual well-being—can the industry position itself as a responsible societal institution with a long-term, profitable future.

The American Society for Healthcare Engineering (ASHE 2001) has explicitly defined a role for the industry in protecting health through its operations and buildings as the core values for sustainable design practices :

- protecting the immediate health of building occupants,
- protecting the health of the surrounding community, and
- protecting the health of the larger global community.

This "triple bottom line for health" defines the industry approach to sustainable building and operations and is the basis for design tools and guidance documents that have been developed to assist healthcare organizations in meeting these challenges. Figure 5.2 illustrates the triple bottom line concept necessary for businesses to succeed in today's socially responsible and environmentally concerned climate. As awareness of the healthcare industry's environmental footprint increases, consumers will demand the same kind of best practices leadership that directs successful corporations (Elkington 1998).

The idea of a triple bottom line dates back to the mid-1990s (SustainAbility and United Nations Environment Programme 2002) and gained popularity with the 1997 publication of the British edition of John Elkington's (1998) *Cannibals with Forks: The Triple Bottom Line of the 21st Century Business*. The triple bottom line concept has been used to describe a framework for measuring and reporting business performance against economic, social, and environmental parameters rather than maximizing profits or growth. Corporations have realized that businesses lacking social and ecological integrity are not economically viable over the long run; their costs eventually increase and customer loyalty declines. In turn they focus on conserving nonrenewable resources and protecting the environment and on being good neighbors and good corporate citizens as means of maintaining long-term profitability.

Improved economic performance, even in the short term, has been realized in many cases when managers pay increased attention to social and ecological performance. They are also finding ways to transform wastes into economic assets for increased production while using fewer costly, nonrenewable resources. Developing and maintaining better relationships with their workers, customers, and others in the communities in which companies operate can lead to reduced labor costs and create new markets (Hawken, Lovins, and Lovins 1999).

Figure 5.2: The Triple Bottom Line for Health

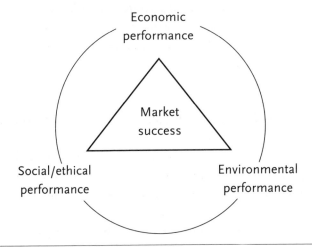

This concept has taken on a number of different labels—green economics, full-cost accounting, natural capital—but could be thought of as just good business. Many CEOs believe that sustainability is vital to the profitability of any company, as evidenced by a PriceWaterhouseCoopers survey (2002) of 1,000 CEOs from 43 countries. Figure 5.2 demonstrates the triple bottom line of socially responsible businesses, which seek to integrate environmental, social, and economic values in their products and services.

The state of California is responsible for a major portion of healthcare construction activity, driven by the need to reconstruct to meet new seismic regulations. Kaiser Permanente, for example, expects to spend upward of $13.1 billion before 2013 on 25 new hospitals, replacements, or significant additions and more than 400 new medical office buildings. To guide this effort Kaiser built on the ASHE Guidance Statement and LEED-NC to develop a customized "eco toolkit" of sustainable building strategies. In 2004 the *Green Guide for Health Care* became the industry's first quantifiable guide to integrating enhanced environmental health principles and practices into the planning, design, construction, and operations of healthcare facilities. The *Green Guide* is a self-certifying metric tool that highlights health-based benefits of sustainable design strategies in site planning, energy and water conservation, materials, and indoor environmental quality. It also includes strategies for improving the environmental performance of existing buildings through operation, with topics ranging from waste management to environmentally preferable purchasing.

Protecting the Immediate Health of Building Occupants

Protecting the immediate health of building occupants begins by designing healing environments to minimize negative impacts on both the physical and psychological health of the occupants—patients and health providers alike. A better building has been defined as one that reduces stress and improves safety for its occupants (Berry et al. 2004). Factors that define indoor environmental quality directly affect occupant health and well-being. Indoor air quality (IAQ) and toxic components of materials can affect the safety and physical well-being of the occupants just as the acoustical environment and connection to the natural world through daylighting and views can reduce stress and positively affect patient outcomes and staff productivity (see Chapter 4).

Indoor Air Quality

IAQ has emerged as a key issue in sustainable design because of its central relationship to occupant health and productivity, energy conservation, building materials, and HVAC system design. Poor IAQ has been linked to sick building syndrome, building-related illnesses, and multiple chemical sensitivities. The U.S. Environmental Protection Agency (EPA) and National Institute of Occupational Safety and Health define good IAQ as including introduction and distribution of adequate ventilation air, control of airborne contaminants, and maintenance of acceptable temperature and relative humidity. A national survey of 415 office workers found that nearly half (49 percent) chose IAQ as the first or second workplace aspect they would like to see improved and linked poor health to poor IAQ resulting in reduced work performance (Opinion Research Corporation 2005).

Studies indicate that most people spend as much as 90 percent of their time indoors and that indoor air levels of many pollutants may be 25 times, and on occasion 100 times, higher than outdoor levels (EPA-AHA 1998). Accordingly, EPA and its science advisory board rank indoor air pollution among the top five environmental risks to public health. It has further been suggested that "improving buildings and indoor environments could reduce health-care and sick leave and increase worker performance, resulting in an estimated productivity gain of $30 to $150 billion annually" (Fisk and Rosenfeld 1997).

Hospitals, despite their high ventilation rates, are in line with other industries in terms of IAQ and worker health. The Joint Commission on Accreditation of Healthcare Organizations recommends that hospitals establish IAQ programs to monitor the increasing risks associated with these issues (Hansen 1997). From 1980 to 1994 reported lung and respiratory claims in California increased by more than 500 percent. In a study on cleaning products and work-related asthma conducted in four states, healthcare workers (including both environmental services and professional staff) accounted for more than 40 percent of adult-onset asthma cases (Rosenman et al. 2003).

Building materials can have a significant impact on IAQ in terms of odors, particles, and volatile organic compounds (VOCs).[1] The most significant sources of VOCs include wet-applied products such as paints, sealers, and adhesives, plus pesticides and joint compounds. Other materials like carpeting, vinyl flooring, wood-sheet products (e.g., particleboard, plywood), insulation, and furnishings likewise emit VOCs. Wet-applied materials are a major concern because they evaporate after application and therefore release a large percentage of their weight. Carpets not only release VOCs, or off-gas, but also act as sinks to absorb VOCs released by other products in close proximity, slowly rereleasing the VOCs over time. Likewise, drywall, acoustical ceiling products, furnishings, and fabrics act as sinks.

Urea-formaldehyde, another off-gassing substance, is used extensively in construction materials, representing 70 percent of its use.

Latex paints, glues, lacquers as well as plywood, particleboard, decorative laminates, and fiberglass insulation all emit urea-formaldehyde, especially when new. Formaldehyde levels are normally much higher indoors than outdoors and are irritating to tissues when they come into direct contact. The most common symptoms include irritation of the eyes, nose, and throat along with increased tearing. The International Agency for Research on Cancer (2004) has concluded that formaldehyde is carcinogenic to humans.

Particles (dusts) and bioaerosols (fungus, bacteria, pollen, mites) are another common contributor to poor IAQ. Installation and maintenance of HVAC systems is a major component in the IAQ equation. These systems must be able to displace VOCs, respired carbon dioxide, body odors, fragrances, skin flakes, and particles shed from clothing and office machines such as copiers and laser printers. Additionally, the systems must provide dehumidification. Because microorganisms need water to grow, moisture intrusion into buildings plays a critical role in sick building issues.

IAQ is a serious subject brought to the forefront of public attention by media reports of legionnaires' disease, salmonella and E. coli bacteria, and other sources of sick buildings and building-related illnesses. Accordingly, one law review reports that more than $700 million in damages have been awarded to date in IAQ lawsuits, with a $1 million average settlement. Aside from the liability exposure, numerous studies have shown that buildings designed for good IAQ have many benefits, including increased production, safety, morale, and general well-being of the occupants, not to mention extended life and value of the building.

Material Resources

The extraction, manufacturing, transportation, use, and disposal of building materials have significant impacts on the environment—the air we breathe, water we drink, and body burden of chemicals we carry. Inevitably, consideration of healthy communities leads to careful consideration of this component of the sustainable building process. Healthcare practitioners recognize that problems can be triggered by exposure to indoor air pollutants, mercury, latex, polyvinyl chloride (PVC), disinfectants, laboratory chemicals, and hundreds of other substances used in the health-care environment. Likewise, while healthcare practitioners and organizations have implemented programs to curb toxic materials in use, they have in many cases overlooked the larger life cycle impacts of the building materials around them and their effect on the healthcare environment.

Persistent bioaccumulative toxins (PBTs) are of particular health concern because they do not break down quickly in the environment and concentrate as they are ingested up the food chain. These toxins have a range of adverse human health effects, including effects on the nervous and reproductive systems, genetic impacts with associated developmental problems, and cancer. Because of their high toxicity and persistent bioaccumulative characteristics, even small, difficult-to-detect releases can lead to harmful exposures. These issues have led to strategies targeting elimination of production and use of substances that are PBTs or are known to lead to their formation, instead of controlling emissions as with VOCs.

Five PBTs commonly addressed in elimination policies have direct links with building materials: cadmium, lead, mercury, dioxins (including furans and dioxin-like compounds), and polychlorinated biphenyls (PCBs). These substances are either used as additives in building materials or produced and released into the environment during the life cycle of the material.

Quantifying the environmental impacts of materials is the goal of life cycle assessment methodologies. Currently, life cycle assessment tools for materials are not developed to account for impacts associated with toxic chemicals. However, healthcare organizations are quick to embrace the notion of, for example, constructing cancer centers without materials containing known or suspected carcinogens. Can we create a framework for more informed, sustainable material choices?

At the forefront of materials transformation, architect William McDonough and chemist Michael Braungart have launched the MBDC Design Protocol, known within the green building industry as "cradle to cradle" thinking. Many manufacturers are rethinking their manufacturing processes to remove harmful chemicals, minimize waste, and conserve resources.

Within the healthcare industry, leading healthcare systems are reconnecting to the "Precautionary Principle" in their approach to chemical and construction: "When an activity raises threats of harm to human health or the environment, precautionary measures should be taken even if some cause and effect relationships are not fully established scientifically" (Science & Environmental Health Network 1998). This principle guides the approach to chemical evaluation and supports the growing number of worldwide industries that are developing and implementing high-hazard-materials screening methodologies.

Connection to the Natural World

As reported in other growing volume of scientific evidence and case studies indicate that environmental factors do affect the quality of healthcare. Connection to nature and lighting form the outdoors (i.e., daylighting) are examples of concepts supported by both evidence-based design research and sustainable building practice. Daylight harvesting also presents a potential benefit of a 50 percent to 80 percent reduction in energy use during the sunlit part of the day (Public Technology 1996).

Energy conservation through daylighting as a sustainable feature can also render therapeutic results. Biochemical and hormonal body rhythms can be influenced by the amount of light exposure, as can the synthesis of certain vitamins (Ulrich 1993). Studies at the University of Michigan (Clay 2001) have found that employees with views of a natural landscape report greater job satisfaction, less stress, and fewer illnesses.

Protecting the Health of the Surrounding Community

The health of a community can be directly affected by choices made and practices followed by its citizens and institutions. Since

Figure 5.3: Applying the Triple Bottom Line Approach at the Community Level

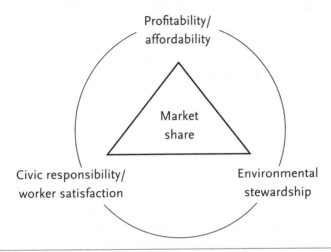

Profitability/
affordability

Market
share

Civic responsibility/
worker satisfaction

Environmental
stewardship

the mid-1990s the healthcare industry has made major strides in expanding its mission to include community health. In the area of operations the healthcare industry is cleaning up its own house, which serves to make healthcare organizations better community health advocates.

In keeping with the 1998 memorandum of understanding between the EPA and American Hospital Association (1998) overall waste reduction, strategies for eliminating incineration, and the elimination of mercury in medical devices are a few examples of steps the industry has taken to be a better neighbor. Operational initiatives such as increased recycling, mercury thermometer take-back programs, introduction of farmers' markets on hospital properties, and surplus food donations to food banks all demonstrate community and public health values. Figure 5.3 illustrates a most compelling reason for hospitals to apply the triple bottom line methodology first at the community scale, where the rate of return for incorporating good-neighbor policies is likely to be highest (Elkington 1998).

The most visible impacts of the built environment on the community arise from land use, utility infrastructure, and transportation decisions. Large institutions potentially burden a community's ability to meet the needs of its citizens if basic planning and infrastructure decisions are not managed wisely. Degradation of local ecosystems and water resources can directly affect the community's long-term health and survival. Sustainable land use and energy practices have the potential to obviate actual and perceived burdens.

Land Use

Sustainable site design examines how local and regional conditions influence and shape the site of a proposed building. Rather than emphasizing the manipulation of the existing landscape to conform to a standard or optimal plan, it engages the design team in proactive analysis of how the site influences the design of the building, with a goal toward enhancing the relationship between the built environment and natural world. Planning a sustainable site encompasses review of natural ecosystems and community resources to minimize the disruption to undeveloped land, habitat, and natural water flows and maximize view-shed opportunities. (A view shed is a physiographic area composed of land, water, biotic, and cultural elements that may be viewed and mapped from one or more viewpoints and that has inherent scenic qualities and/or aesthetic values as determined by those who view it.) Sustainable site planning seeks to amplify the benefits from building orientation and the site's natural features so that the improvement resonates past the property boundary.

Consideration is also given to returning brownfield sites—land once used for other purposes, often industrial or commercial site where expansion or redevelopment is complicated by real or perceived environmental contamination—productive economic use by mitigating the negative impact on human and environmental health. As urbanism continues to evolve and the density of our cities increases, the utilization of brownfield sites becomes an increasingly valuable asset to the community.

Transportation

It has long been recognized by both science and government that air quality has a direct impact on health and that fossil, fuel-burning vehicles directly affect air quality. These impacts include vehicle emissions that contribute to smog and air pollution in addition to environmental damage from oil extraction and refining. There are few environmentally benign alternatives to fossil-fueled transportation; however, alternative practices and policies exist that, combined with other strategies, can reduce community impacts and improve air quality.

Healthcare organizations are finding that by restricting the size of parking lots, promoting carpooling activities, and working with community transportation authorities to improve access to public transportation, benefits to community and human health can be achieved. As healthcare campuses become denser and the resulting loss of green space becomes more acute, reduction of parking lots and structures appears more promising in solving land-use issues in addition to reducing other community burdens such as storm water runoff and the urban heat island effect, which occur when warmer temperatures are experienced in urban landscape compared to adjacent rural areas as a result of solar energy retention on constructed surfaces.

When convenient alternatives such as bicycles, mass transportation, and carpooling are available, a surprisingly large number of patients and staff are willing to take advantage of these less costly modes of transportation. With fuel costs continuing to climb, more people are finding it more difficult to justify high personal transportation expenses and are looking for alternatives.

Large healthcare organizations have other cleaner transportation choices that many smaller organizations may not. These larger organizations typically operate fleets of vehicles for the purposes of serving, maintaining, and operating their facilities. These vehicles range from ambulances to delivery vans to shuttle buses, which often operate continuously and relatively locally. By reducing emissions, alternative-fuel and fuel-efficient fleets demonstrate a clear commitment to the health of building occupants and the surrounding community, often while reducing operating expenses.

Community infrastructures for water, sanitary, and storm sewers are rapidly aging while new capacity demands accelerate this deterioration. As the demand grows, many communities find it more difficult to upgrade and expand their infrastructures because of overextended fiscal budgets. While growth in community institutions is good for the tax base and job creation, the tax-exempt status of many healthcare organizations only makes the issue worse because tax dollars are not accessed on the increased property values resulting from facility expansions. Responsible healthcare organizations can ease their burdens on community infrastructures by instituting water-conservation policies, on-site stormwater management programs, and reduced sewage discharges through efficient water use.

As industry accounts for 16 percent of the world's water consumption, the amount of fresh water consumed by buildings and their landscape irrigation systems is a key concern of sustainable design. U.S. hospitals typically use 80 to 150 gallons of water per bed per day (Bristol Meyers Squibb 2004). Water use in hospitals breaks down into three major categories: irrigation, potable uses in which high-quality water is essential (e.g., hand washing, showers, sewage conveyance), and process uses in which water is used for industrial applications (e.g., cooling tower makeup, coolant, sterile processing, food service). In an average mid-sized acute care hospital, more than 70 percent of the water use is for process applications (Mouratore 2002). Sustainable design practice reduces water demands through three strategies: (1) reducing or eliminating potable water use for landscape irrigation, (2) reducing potable water use through high-efficiency fixtures, and (3) substituting potable water use in process water applications.

Already water shortages in the West and Midwest are demanding conservation efforts. Sustainable design can answer these demands by reducing consumption of fresh water through specification of materials that do not waste water in their manufacture, selection of water-efficient fixtures and appliances, and selection of landscape vegetation that requires minimum irrigation. More advanced designs can implement graywater and rainwater harvesting systems for sewage conveyance and irrigation.

Waste Management

"Source reduction is to garbage what preventive medicine is to health—a means of avoiding trouble before it happens" (Rathje and Murphy 2001). Trouble in waste disposal is fast approaching. The number of U.S. landfills decreased from 20,000 in 1978 to just over 3,000 by 2002 and is estimated by the EPA to be fewer than 1,300 by 2008. But the tipping fees—the cost for dumping a load of waste into a given landfill—and volume of nonhazardous waste continue to increase, reaching 409 million tons in 2001, almost double that in 1990. Construction and demolition waste accounts for more than 35 percent of that volume, requiring several states (e.g., Massachusetts, Florida, and California) to impose mandatory construction and demolition waste recycling to slow demands on the ever-diminishing landfill space.

Healthcare organizations average between 70 million and 75 million square feet of construction annually. Typical construction projects generate approximately 2.2 pounds of waste per square foot, or 77,000 to 82,500 tons of construction waste a year. Projects that recycle construction and demolition debris may benefit from the cost synergies and trade-offs of reduced tipping fees and hauling charges. Many organizations have actually realized a profit from construction waste management programs. Diversion of the construction and demolition waste stream through salvaging and recycling can contribute to extending the life of existing community landfills, while reducing the demand for virgin resources and easing community opposition to expanding landfills.

Watershed Protection

The quality of a community's water resources directly affects public health and its ability to grow and prosper. Shortage of water, as addressed earlier, is just one of the water issues many communities face; the quality of that water directly determines how that resource can be used safely. Both air quality and the condition of the watershed affect a water source's quality. As every building site is in a watershed, activities on a site have a direct impact on that watershed's condition. These activities, both during and after construction, can destroy aquatic life and pollute water supplies. Construction can intensify soil erosion, causing sedimentation of waterways and aggravating flooding. Roadways and parking lots can pollute water resources with runoff of hydrocarbons (oil, gasoline, diesel) and chemicals (antifreeze, de-icing salts). Runoff from overmaintained landscapes can rob soils of nutrients while discharging fertilizers, herbicides, and pesticides into the watershed.

Watershed protection through erosion and sedimentation control, low-maintenance native landscapes, and rainwater harvesting contributes to the health of the ecosystem and water resources. Working with a site's natural systems can contribute to preserving and restoring a healthy watershed and the community it supports.

Protecting the Health of the Global Community

As community choices and practices can affect the immediate community, so too can their accumulated affects determine the planet's ability to sustain current and future generations. Although the growth rate has slowed, the population is still expected to reach 9 billion by 2050, placing increasing demands on the environment and its ability to sustain us. There is no longer any debate by the scientific community that global warming is not only real but man-made and presents perhaps humanity's greatest challenge (Headden 2004).

Climate Change and Air Quality

Building energy use is responsible for at least 30 percent of U.S. greenhouse gas releases into the atmosphere, a precursor to global warming (Department of Energy 1999). When we add the gaseous releases associated with building materials extraction, production, and transportation, totals increase to more than 40 percent. Additionally, buildings contribute to the depletion of the stratospheric ozone layer by using refrigerants and products, including some insulation materials, manufactured with ozone-depleting compounds such as chlorofluorocarbons (CFCs). The world community has recognized the importance of ozone depletion, and 160 countries signed the Montreal Protocol on Substances that Deplete the Ozone Layer in 1987.

In 1996 the EPA identified dioxin as the most potent human carcinogen ever measured and named medical waste incineration as the major source of dioxin emissions in the United States. Since then the industry has dramatically decreased reliance on incineration: the number of medical waste incinerators in North America has decreased from 5,600 in 1996 to just under 100 (Health Care Without Harm 2005). Atmospheric dioxin levels reached a peak in the mid-1990s and are now declining. This has been accomplished through the combined strategies of water reduction, increased alternative water treatment technologies, and avoidance of chlorinated products in the incineration waste system.

Energy Efficiency

Buildings use 40 percent of the nation's energy. The healthcare sector is responsible for 11 percent of all commercial consumption, using a total of 561 trillion BTUs (Energy Information Administration 1995). The political and environmental consequences of continued dependence on fossil fuels are well-documented. Moreover, the use of fossil fuels for energy production has direct or indirect consequences for human health. Improving energy efficiency is the best way to meet energy demands without adding to air and water pollution.

Until now the answer to improved indoor air quality has been increased ventilation rates. However, as recently as 1997 estimates were that a 10 percent increase in ventilation rates equated to an increase of 33 percent in energy consumption. Today, with energy costs exceed 50 percent of many plant operations budgets it is no longer viable to simply increase ventilation rates without consideration of the impact on operational dollars. Instead, there is renewed focus on heat recovery technologies (where heat from air being exhausted is "recovered" by the incoming fresh air, without cross contamination of the actual air stream). Effort on reducing indoor air pollutants may begin to affect the need for increased air exchanges. Many states and municipalities are instituting rebates or incentives to encourage building owners to pursue technologies that reduce energy demand in buildings. EPA's Energy Star for Healthcare is a partnership program that many institutions have turned to assess and manage their energy usage. The program collects actual energy usage data from the facility and established a baseline rating. The rating then allows the facility to prioritize its energy investments, set goals, and track management success.

Nature

Climate change resulting from global warming is also expected to increase the spread of disease vectors far from their current regions, destabilizing ecosystems and threatening worldwide nutrition. Warmer weather would affect transmission of insect-borne diseases such as malaria and West Nile virus.

Loss of rainforests from unsustainable forest management can result in the loss of medicines and irreplaceable genetic information that could lead to new medical breakthroughs. It's now believed that the biggest value of stable forests may be in storing carbon, carbon that would be released as greenhouse gases by burning from clearing practices for agriculture and development.

THE TRIPLE BOTTOM LINE FOR PERFORMANCE

As a largely not-for-profit sector, developing a business case for sustainability in healthcare must begin with the understanding that the industry is always engaged in triple bottom line accounting. Often, healthcare service lines are developed and continued despite poor economic performance for the sake of social goals. Healthcare executives often use the concept of "margin into mission" to describe this reality.

Figure 5.4: The Integral Framework of Socially Responsible Organizations

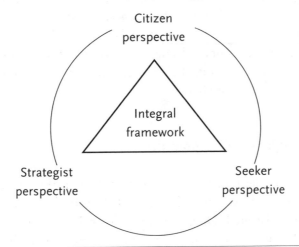

The integral way suggests a structural framework for creating perspective and the governing principles for personal decision making. The seeker governs environmental performance, the citizen social values, and the strategist economic outcome. Private for-profit businesses traditionally emphasizes economic performance—socially responsible models seek a more balanced framework. A useful construct for examining this business case, termed the *integral way*, define three distinct perspectives: the seeker is concerned with environmental performance, the citizen with social performance, and the strategist with economic performance. Figure 5.4 illustrates the interplay among the seeker, citizen, and strategist perspectives. The integral way suggests a structural framework for creating perspective and the governing principals for personal decision making. The seeker governs environmental performance; the citizen, social values; and the strategist, economic outcome (Frankel 2004).

In healthcare organizations each of these viewpoints combines to provide a complex decision-making structure that attempts to balance multiple priorities and viewpoints. Figure 5.5 applies the integral framework to healthcare decision makers. Governing principles for the healthcare sector and its margin-to-mission reality are more complex and multidimensional than simple economic accounting might suggest, as the various administrative roles participate in defining business success. A unique business case is defined for each: an economic business case for the strategist, a social business case for the citizen, and a visionary leadership business case for the seeker. Ultimately, these individual business case threads weave together to form a unified case for change.

The Strategist Case: Economics

The most prevalent notion in the market today is that green buildings cost more. First, the question, "Cost more than what?" must be carefully answered. Do green buildings cost more than the exact same building without the green features, more than the capital budget, or more than comparable buildings of the same size and complexity? In the absence of green buildings to study, financial models have predicted that sustainable buildings would carry cost premiums related to their level of sustainability.

The Packard Foundation (2002) considered the construction and operations costs associated with its own proposed Los Altos, California, office building and concluded that construction costs would increase with the level of achievement, reaching a premium of 30 percent for a living building (i.e., a building that produced its own power and treated the wastes generated on site), whereas long-term ownership costs (including operation) would fall by 15 percent per year for the building's life span. Based on the results of this study the Foundation recommended an aggressive green building program.

More recent studies based on completed buildings have shown that the anticipated cost premiums have been largely overstated. In a white paper on sustainability an editor at *Building Design and Construction* magazine concluded that many green buildings cost no more than their brown equivalents (Cassidy 2003). Kats (2003) reviewed more than 100 completed LEED-certified office and school buildings and concluded that the average first-cost premium was slightly less than 2 percent. More importantly these studies point to a consistent set of key factors that affects building costs:

Figure 5.5: The Integral Framework Applied to Healthcare Decision Makers

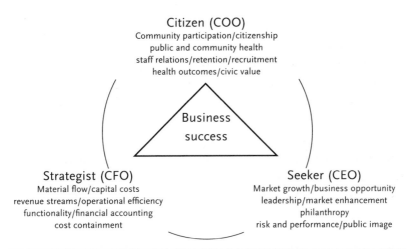

Citizen (COO)
Community participation/citizenship
public and community health
staff relations/retention/recruitment
health outcomes/civic value

Business
success

Strategist (CFO)
Material flow/capital costs
revenue streams/operational efficiency
functionality/financial accounting
cost containment

Seeker (CEO)
Market growth/business opportunity
leadership/market enhancement
philanthropy
risk and performance/public image

- The earlier the green features are incorporated into the design, the lower the cost.
- Costs decline with increasing experience and as market transformation occurs.
- Green buildings provide financial benefits that brown buildings do not.

Kats (2003) outlined these benefits as follows: "The financial benefits are in lower operating costs, lower environmental costs, and increased productivity and health. Over 20 years, the benefits are over 10 times the additional costs." Matthiessen and Morris (2004) concluded: "Sustainability is a program issue rather than an added requirement; perhaps the most important thing to remember is that . . . [it] is not a below the line item." That study, which compared completed green and brown laboratory buildings, found no correlation between construction cost and level of sustainable design features. Instead, it concluded:

- Great variation exists in costs of buildings, even within the same building program type.
- There are low- and high-cost green buildings; there are low- and high-cost brown buildings.

There are no conclusive data that in the aggregate green buildings cost more than their brown equivalents. If green strategies that cost more than their brown equivalents but deliver operational savings are isolated, the operational savings must find their way into the equation. Examples of such operational savings include energy and water efficiency savings or material selections that reduce maintenance costs. The EPA estimates that every dollar saved in operation is equivalent to $20 in new revenue (Reed 2000).

The Citizen Case: Social Value of Sustainable Building

At the same time the strategist deals with the financial implications, the citizen reviews the social implications of sustainable building practices (see Figure 5.5). The citizen prioritizes the relationship between buildings and health. It is in this realm that the intersection with evidence-based design is most evident. As Chapter 7 illustrates, there is financial payback in constructing buildings that reduce stress and improve safety. Often, additional organizational social benefit is achieved through an integrated design process that engages a wide group of stakeholders, where the building design is viewed as only one component of an institutionwide environmental improvement initiative that involves everyone. As Lance Secretan (2005) put it: "There is no actual nursing shortage. There is a shortage of places that nurses want to work."

Defining organizational and community benefits that arise from sustainable building strategies is the current challenge in healthcare. These benefits need to be defined, quantified, and communicated through industry, much the way the Fable Hospital example presented in Chapter 7 provides important initial data to use in quantification of benefits such as staff illness and absenteeism, improved staff performance (reduced medical errors), reduced hospital-acquired infections, and improved staff recruitment and retention.

At the same time hospitals have realized that enormous social benefit accrues from implementing improved environmental performance strategies through operations. Whether organizations receive recognition for recycling programs, reductions in medical waste incineration, or implementation of farmers' markets on site, environmental improvement programs resonate with communities. To date, many of the sustainable healthcare projects have engaged in sustainable design to reduce both real and perceived community impacts from their development footprint. Some municipalities have instituted expedited approval processes for LEED projects, particularly for sites with drainage and water management challenges.

The Seeker Case: Environmental Leadership

Until there are enough green healthcare buildings to study and the business case is proven, sustainable healthcare construction will be accomplished by a select group of industry leaders. Why do healthcare organizations strive to be leaders in this area? They do it to enhance their community and medical reputations; improve staff recruitment and retention; and increase market share, philanthropy, and research grants. Each of these considerations is directly affected by sustainable building practices.

In 2003 the Kresge Foundation launched a Green Building Initiative, becoming the first major philanthropic organization to commit to exclusively fund green building. Sustainable building resonates with an increasing number of private donors and board members, particularly as the private business sector accelerates green building tax credit programs and other market-based incentives. Likewise, ecological medicine is moving into medical and nursing school curricula, which will soon affect incoming medical professionals.

CONCLUSION

Can healthcare organizations afford to build green? A better question may be whether they can afford not to. In *The Tipping Point* Malcolm Gladwell (2000) describes three requirements that must be met to create an environment in which a new idea can inexorably take hold, when a tipping point is reached. First, there is the wisdom of the few. In the healthcare market nearly 100 LEED and Green Guide Pilot projects along with 5,000 Green Guide registrants more than meet this challenge. Second, there is the stickiness factor—that is, the elements in place to sustain a new trend. The 2006 *AIA* (American Institute of Architects and Facility Guidelines Institute) *Guidelines for Design and Construction of Hospital and Healthcare Facilities Healthcare Construction* include references to sustainable and evidence-based design practice, and an increasing number of state and local governments are requiring building design to meet LEED requirements. Third, Gladwell (2000) describes the power of context. For healthcare the compelling links between buildings and health, the irony of a healthcare system that may contribute to environmental illness, and the strong connection to healthcare's fundamental mission to "first, do no harm" make sustainable building an important goal that is impossible to ignore.

NOTE

1. The term volatile organic compounds (VOCs) refers collectively to a large number of mostly petrochemical-derived substrates that readily volatize, or become a breathable gas, at room temperature and therefore contaminate indoor air. VOCs in the atmosphere react with oxides of nitrogen in the presence of sunlight, forming ground-level ozone that is a major component of smog. Exposure to ground-level ozone is associated with a wide variety of human health effects, with respiratory afflictions being one of the more serious health hazards. Those with preexisting respiratory disease are at increased risk.

REFERENCES

American Institute of Architects and Facility Guidelines Institute. Forthcoming. *Guidelines for the Design and Construction of Hospital and Healthcare Facilities.* Washington, DC.

American Society for Healthcare Engineering. 2001. *The Green Healthcare Construction Guidance Statement.* Chicago: ASHE.

American Society of Healthcare Environmental Services. 1993. *An Ounce of Prevention.* Chicago: ASHES.

Berry, L., D. Parker, R. Coile, D. K. Hamilton, D. O'Neill, and B. Sadler. 2004. "The Business Case for Better Buildings." *Frontiers of Health Services Management* (21) 1: 3–24.

Bristol Meyers Squibb. 2004. *Greener Hospitals: Improving Environmental Performance,* edited by the Environmental Science Center. Augsburg, Germany: Bristol Meyers Squibb.

Clay, R. 2001. "Green Is Good for You." *Monitor on Psychology* (32) 4. [Online article; retrieved 4/17/01.]

Cassidy, R. 2003. "White Paper on Sustainability." *Building Design and Construction Magazine,* November 1.

Dean, L. 2000. "Setting Healthcare's Environmental Agenda," Society of Healthcare Epidemiology of America conference proceedings, San Francisco, October 16–18.

Elkington, J. 1998. *Cannibals with Forks: The Triple Bottom Line of 21st Century Business.* Oxford, UK: Capstone Publishing.

Energy Information Administration. 1996. *Commercial Building Energy Consumption Survey.* Washington, DC: EIA.

EPA-AHA. 1998. "United States Environmental Protection Agency (EPA) and the American Hospital Association (AHA) Memorandum of Understanding." [Online information; retrieved 08/21/05.] www.h2e-online.org/about/mov.htm.

Fisk, W., and A. osenfeld. 1997. "Improved Productivity and Health from Better Indoor Environments." *Center for Building Science Newsletter* #15 Summer: 5.

Frankel, C. 2004. *Out of the Labyrinth.* Reinbeck, NY: Monkfish Book Publishing.

Gladwell, M. 2000. *The Tipping Point: How Little Things Can Make a Big Difference.* New York: Little, Brown and Co.

Hansen, W. 1997. *A Guide to Managing Indoor Air Quality in Healthcare Organizations.* Oakbrook Terrace, IL: Joint Commission on Accreditation of Healthcare Organizations.

Hawken, P., A. Lovins, and L. H. Lovins. 1999. *Natural Capitalism.* New York: Little, Brown and Co.

Headden, S. (ed.). 2004. "A Heavy Footprint." *U.S. News & World Report* Special Edition, 5.

Health Care Without Harm. 2005. "Stericycle Burns Waste and Endangers Shareholder Investments, Communities' Health." [Online press release; retrieved 04/29/05.] www.noharm.org/details.cfm?type=document&id=1067.

International Agency for Research on Cancer. 2004. "IARC Classified Formaldehyde as Carcinogenic to Humans." Press release no. 153. Lyon, France, June.

Kats, G. 2003. "Green Building Costs and Financial Benefits." [Online article.] www.cap-e.com.

Lawrence, D. 2000. "Setting Healthcare's Environmental Agenda." Society of Healthcare Epidemiology of America conference proceedings, San Francisco, October 21, 1966.

Lerner, M. 2000. "Setting Healthcare's Environmental Agenda." Presentation at Society of Healthcare Epidemiology of America conference, San Francisco, October.

Lounsbury, M. 2003. "On Location: GreenBuild 2003." *Sustainable Industries Journal*. [Online article retrieved 05/15/04.] www.greenerbuildings.com/news _detail.cfm?NewsID=26214.

Matthiessen, L. F., and P. Morris. 2004. "Costing Green: A Comprehensive Cost Database and Budgeting Methodology." [Online document; retrieved 08/21/05.] www.greenerbuildings.com.

Mouratore, T. 2002. "Benchmarking Best Practices in Water Conservation." Presentation at ASHE 39th Annual Conference and Technology Exhibition, Nashville, Tennessee. July 29–31.

National Center for Health Statistics, Centers for Disease Control and Prevention. 1998. "Hospital Utilization and Expenditures." [Online information; retrieved 07/09/01.] www.cdc.gov/nchs/fastats/hospital.htm.

Opinion Research Corporation. 2005. "Workers Want Better IAQ." *Consulting-Specifying Engineer,* April 15.

The Packard Foundation. 2002. *Building for Sustainability Report: Six Scenarios for the David and Lucille Packard Los Altos Project*. Palo Alto, CA: Packard Foundation.

PricewaterhouseCoopers. 2002. "Sustainability Survey Report." August. [Online information; retrieved 05/15/05.] www.pwcglobal.com.

Public Technology, Inc. 1996. *Sustainable Building Technical Manual.* Washington, DC: Public Technology, Inc.

Rathje, W., and C. Murphy. 2001. *Rubbish! The Archaeology of Garbage.* Tucson, AZ: University of Arizona Press.

Reed, C. 2000. *U.S. Environmental Protection Agency Research of Energy Star Hospital Partners.* Unpublished data.

Rosenman, K., M. J. Reilly, D. P. Schill, D. Vallante, J. Flattery, R. Harrison, F. Reinish, E. Pechter, L. Davis, C. M. Tumpowsky, and M. Filios. 2003. "Cleaning Products and Work Related Asthma." *Journal of Occupational and Environmental Medicine* 45 (5): 556–63.

Science & Environmental Health Network. 1998. "Precautionary Principle." Presentation at Wingspread Conference on the Precautionary Principle, Racine, Wisconsin, January 26. [Online article; retrieved 06/01/05.] www.sehn.org/wing.html.

Secretan, L. 2005. "Reclaiming Higher Ground." Presentation at EnvironDesign 9, New York, April 19.

SustainAbility Ltd. and United Nations Environment Programme. 2002. *Trust Us: The Global Reporters 2002 Survey of Corporate Sustainability Reporting.* London: SustainAbility LTD.

U.S. Department of Energy, Energy Information Administration. 1999. *Emissions of Greenhouse Gases in the United States 1999.* Washington, DC: DOE.

U.S. Environmental Protection Agency. 1998. "A Comparison of Indoor and Outdoor Concentrations of Hazardous Air Pollutants." *Inside IAQ* (Spring/Summer): 1–7.

Ulrich, R. 1993. "Biophilia, Biophobia, and Natural Landscapes." In *The Biophilia Hypothesis*, edited by E. O. Wilson. Washington, DC: Island Press.

CHAPTER 6

Designing a Better Environment

Jain Malkin

MUCH HAS BEEN written in the past 15 years about healing environments. Indeed, the term has even been used to anoint programs to update interior finishes in a nursing unit. Increasingly, hospitals have been sending out requests for proposals (RFPs) for architectural services requiring design professionals to demonstrate proficiency in this area, but at the time of the interview no one knows the right questions to ask. The healing environment is treated as if it were a commodity that could be bought merely by issuing an RFP. If only it were that simple.

The research on healing environments falls roughly into five categories: (1) connection to nature, (2) options and choices, (3) access to social support, (4) elimination of environmental stressers, and (5) positive diversions. Overall, a healing environment is one that is psychologically supportive for patients, their families, and for staff. The essential triad for creating a healing environment is evidence-based design, operational performance, and organizational culture. To address any one of these components without the other would be analogous to building a two-legged stool. It would be unbalanced.

HISTORICAL ORIGINS

The Planetree Model Hospital Project in San Francisco in the mid-1980s challenged the very essence of what it means to deliver care in a way that honors and respects the patient. Planetree has had an epic influence on the healthcare industry, culminating in the patient-centered care movement, the first real change in the way care is delivered since 1900. It is difficult to believe that just a handful of passionate contrarians could kick off a revolution in an industry as large as healthcare.

The Nine Elements of Planetree Patient-Centered Care

1. the importance of human interaction,
2. informing and empowering diverse populations (consumer health libraries and patient education),
3. healing partnerships (the importance of including family and friends),
4. nutrition (the nurturing aspects of food),
5. spirituality (inner resources for healing),
6. human touch (the essentials of communicating caring through massage),
7. healing arts (nutrition for the soul),
8. integrating complementary and alternative practices into conventional care, and
9. healing environments (architecture and design conducive to health) (Frampton, Gilpin, and Charmel 2003).

Neurophysiology: Tapping into the Body's Own Pharmacopoeia

One of the most thought-provoking and insightful articles on healing and healing environments was written by a visionary CEO, Patrick Linton (1992), whose originality of thought defined and laid the foundation for a care delivery model that would tap into the "tremendously powerful healing potentials within each human being." Linton based his ideas on the research being done in psychoneuroimmunology, which he explains in a lucid manner in the aforementioned article. Because this research is fundamental to understanding the science behind the intuitive notions people have about why certain types of environments are healing, a summary of observations follows; most are from Linton (1992), and others are noted.

1. The brain, nervous and endocrine systems, and immune system are constantly interacting in a dynamic way. To paraphrase neuroscientist Candace Pert (1997), "These systems are constantly having conversations with each other . . . what you are thinking at any moment is changing your biochemistry."

2. Negative emotions may manifest as a physical disease, whereas positive emotions may positively affect one's health and have, in a variety of studies on cancer patients, been noted to have reduced tumor growth; slowed the progression of the disease; increased natural killer- and T-cell activity; and increased antibody production. Several large studies have found that happiness was a better predictor of future coronary problems than any other clinical variable (Lemonick 2005; Rabin 1999).

3. The brain and nervous system produce neurotransmitter cells that fit receptor cells like a lock and key. This connection engages the immune system. The same thing works in reverse. When the brain is engaged, it produces exactly the right "pharmaceuticals" needed and gets them to the correct place in the precise dosage needed.

Applying psychoneuroimmunology to the effect of the built environment on a patient's experience of stress, neuroscientists have been able to document which areas of the brain are affected by the perception of a healing environment, a setting that feels comfortable or provides pleasure. A pleasant environment keeps norepinephrine levels low so that patients actually experience less pain and have more restful sleep, less anger, less muscle tension, and lower risk of stroke (Rabin 2004). The other major stress hormone, cortisol, can actually damage neurons in the hippocampus and also affects the rate of wound healing. Elevated levels of norepinephrine and cortisol impair the immune system (Rabin 1999).

A Culture of Caring

Although there is an esthetic component associated with a healing environment, it is not tied to a specific style or lavish use of materials. In fact, realization of such an environment can be accomplished on a modest budget. The important element is that patients are able to feel comfortable and that the setting is nonthreatening. A healing environment grows out of a culture of caring in which patient comfort and convenience are priorities. When staff members have this attitude—when they really believe that they are there to serve the patient—they will make decisions on a daily basis that protect and nurture patients.

One cannot underestimate the power of the nurse as an enabler to give the patient confidence and start the healing process. The nurse is often a life raft for the patient—a teacher and guide through the morass of illness to the safety of the riverbank on the other side. This is not to say that every person will be cured or have a good result, but every patient has the potential to be healed in the sense of acceptance of one's condition or limitations and having balance restored—an opportunity to feel whole, to experience the unity of mind, body, and spirit.

THE POWER OF THE BUILT ENVIRONMENT

Just as a caregiver has the ability to help the patient restore balance, the built environment has the potential to be therapeutic. The environment can be an adjunct to clinical care if properly designed to be psychologically supportive, which means that it reduces stress in many dimensions for patients, families, and staff. The concept of a healing environment has evolved in recent years to what is now referred to as evidence-based design. This approach lends more rigor to the research and satisfies those who desire metrics before committing to financial expenditures.

A sizeable body of evidence—some 700 studies—published in peer-reviewed journals offers much guidance in basically three areas: safety, reduction of stress, and ecological health, all of which can and should be used to inform design decisions (Ulrich and Zimring 2004). But it must be said that a building can be designed taking all of this into account and yet be esthetically unappealing and lacking in warmth, comfort, and harmony. There is no substitute for the intuition of a gifted architect or designer or the sheer poetry of great architecture. Within the confines of this chapter, what follows is not a recipe for creating visual poetry but rather a discussion of interior design elements that can make a huge difference in the facility's ambience if skillfully manipulated. Interior finishes must have a nuts-and-bolts practicality for durability and ease of maintenance, but today an array of options score high marks esthetically; many are environmentally friendly as well.

Space Planning and Wayfinding

Space planning should be a collaborative effort between architect and interior designer. As wayfinding legibility is basically a function of good space planning, it is essential to step back and look at the building form and schematic layout to see if architectural landmarks (e.g., a view of a garden, courtyard, or perhaps another building on the campus that has a memorable presence) that can serve as visual cues are present.

A clear strategy should be developed for moving patients from each point of entry to all major destinations. For example, maintaining contact with the outdoors is desirable for all main artery corridors if site planning allows for this. Architectural features such as skylights, atriums, a ceremonial stair, unique public art, and sufficient reinforcements to let people know that they are on the right path become a network of wayfinding aids. These are complemented by artwork and signage and a careful application of color that enhances, but does not compete with, visual wayfinding cues (Malkin 1992). If space planning is well-executed, you should not have to rely on a lot of signage.

Particular attention should be paid to wayfinding issues in parking structures, especially with respect to calling attention to building entries. It is shocking to note how many medical centers fall short in this regard and cause enormous stress for patients and visitors. Likewise, building entries should be obvious and architecturally attention getting for anyone entering the site.

Lighting

Lighting—both natural and electric—is the most important component of an interior environment. Adequate exposure to natural light is essential for biological health and entrainment of circadian rhythms. As discussed in Chapter 4, research indicates that patients in rooms that receive more sunlight are less depressed and have reduced lengths of stay (Ulrich and Zimring 2004). Likewise, staff members who have exposure to natural light may be less fatigued and more able to focus their attention (Tennessen and Cimprich 1995).

Huge, dense buildings that have historically been associated with large medical centers are now being more imaginatively designed to bring light into their cores. In fact, in several European countries every room occupied by humans must have natural light. This does pose a challenge for large buildings, spreading them out horizontally, but it can be done if this is a cultural or code-imposed imperative.

Good lighting design is an art in any building, no less so in hospitals. Indirect lighting should be used in any area where patients are lying on their backs, which means corridors, procedure rooms, and patient rooms. Indirect lighting comes in a variety of forms, from a linear uplighted valance running along the perimeter of a corridor to a recessed cove light or a lay-in light fixture with a reflector that directs the light upward. These fixtures work well for ambient lighting (general illumination) in emergency department treatment rooms, diagnostic imaging rooms, and patient rooms when complemented by examination lights. The standard two-by-four-foot fluorescent fixture with prismatic acrylic lens that has been the hallmark of institutional lighting should be used only in back-of-the-house areas.

Following are a few lighting tips:

- Make use of natural light by way of sidelights alongside doors, skylights, clerestories, and windows whenever possible.
- Use energy-efficient low-mercury content lamps made by manufacturers committed to the Environmental Protection Agency's goals of reduce, reuse, and recycle. The newest lamps provide more lumen output per watt without sacrificing color or ambience.
- Use fluorescent lamps with 3,500-Kelvin color temperature (this refers to the phosphors that coat the lamps) to render colors more realistically and enhance skin tone. Another important dimension of lamp selection is a color-rendering index, or CRI, which should be a minimum of 86 regardless of color temperature. Although it is true that cool-white lamps are less expensive, the gray-blue color they cast on skin tone and interiors makes them a poor investment.
- Use a variety of light fixtures to add design interest.

Ceilings and Acoustics

A wide array of prefabricated ceiling systems offer designers an opportunity to create unique design treatments at far less expense than a custom design. These include a variety of wood ceilings, undulating acrylic panels, aluminum grids, and more. Often, these treatments are combined with acoustical tile. A most important consideration is the noise reduction coefficient (NRC) rating of the tile. Most hospitals and commercial buildings use .65 NRC, which is not adequate to reduce the noise and reverberation in nurses' stations, corridors, and patient rooms. The maximum NRC currently available in acoustical tile is .95, which means that it absorbs 95 percent of the sound energy incident on it. Acoustical tile should be carefully selected for each functional area of the hospital as opposed to using one general tile throughout.

The patient's experience can be enhanced by the placement of images of nature on the ceiling in procedure rooms, such as radiation therapy, diagnostic imaging, endoscopy, and prep and recovery rooms as well as corridors with gurney traffic. These are realistic images printed on film transparencies that are applied to a rigid translucent lens that replaces the standard light fixture lens. Sources for this type of product are The Sky Factory and Art Research Institute.

Color

Do not fear color. A robust application of color by a skilled designer can enliven a space. For many years white walls and floors and corridors that seemed to run to infinity with no accent walls to break the monotony have been synonymous with institutional environments. It is what would come to mind when you pictured a hospital. In recent years, however, architects and designers have embraced color and texture in healthcare settings and used innovative lighting techniques to highlight those features. Children's hospitals today are wonderful examples of design that lifts the spirit, harnessing technology, color, and artwork to delight and educate children. For a thorough discussion of color research specifically for healthcare, see Malkin (2002).

Artwork, Nature, and Music

Works of art are a positive diversion in healthcare settings, enabling patients who are in pain or experiencing anxiety to momentarily take their minds off their problems. In this setting, however, the specific subject matter of the art is important. Roger Ulrich at Texas A&M University states that a person who is ill will interpret a piece of art in a very different way than a person who is well. This is known as the emotional congruence theory—the notion that a person's emotional state can bias the perception of environmental stimuli to match his or her feelings (Bower 1981; Singer and Salovey 1988; Niedenthal, Setterlund, and Jones 1994.)

This means that images that are ambiguous can be frightening, stimulating patients to see hands about to grab them or a sky opening up to swallow them. A scene with an empty chair or a boat dock with an empty boat will, to a healthy person, perhaps recall pleasant memories of a vacation escape, but to a person whose spouse is critically ill the empty chair can symbolize death or abandonment. In a similar vein, artful photographs of women who have had mastectomies may be cathartic for the women who posed for the photos or for the photographer, who might have grappled with recovery from cancer. However, for women about to undergo cancer treatment, exposure to such images can be painful unless they are introduced in a one-on-one session by a therapist who can gauge the readiness of the patient.

Evolutionary theory indicates that images of nature are the most successful in being restorative—relieving stress—for diverse groups of people, provided the subject matter realistically depicts nature, whether it is a view of gardens, water features, mountains, or sand dunes. Compositions that have a depth of perspective and an element of mystery (e.g., a path that winds back into the image, leading the eye to imagine something just around the bend) are especially effective in reducing stress. The research also shows that abstract art can be almost pathological for patients in a treatment or patient care setting; however, this type of art could be considered for lobbies (Ulrich and Lunden 1993; Wypijewski 1997).

Author's Note: For a thoroughly research-based discussion of art in the healthcare setting, see Chapter 7 in *Putting Patients First* by Frampton, Gilpin and Charmel (2003).

Connecting Patients to Nature

An optimal solution for enabling patients to connect with nature in their rooms is by way of a large flat-screen TV and programs such as the Continuous Ambient Relaxation Environment (CARE) Channel.

A disk with 60 hours of nonrepetitive nature images, accompanied by specially composed music based on research as to what is soothing or healing, is provided on a closed-circuit channel through the hospital's network. It can be set as the default whenever someone turns on the TV. A patient may select a specific nature image that will personally be most healing and actually keep it on the screen as a piece of artwork as long as desired or allow the images to sequence. This system was developed for hospitals to provide an alternative to the noise of monitors and conversations overheard from nurses' stations. Built in is a 24-hour clock that adjusts the tempo of the music for nighttime vigils in the intensive care unit, for example, when TV with its annoying advertisements can be stressful for families.

Shaping the Environment with Music

Another system to improve the typical hospital soundscape, developed by Don Campbell, author of *The Mozart Effect*, offers a vast library of world music tailored to the unique function of each area of the hospital from the chapel to the emergency department. Campbell's strategy separates the hospital into unique harmonic zones, each with music of a different tempo and rhythm depending on function and time of day.

Creating a Personal Experience

The Philips Lighting "ambient experience" is designed to allow patients to customize a diagnostic imaging room or even a patient room by waving a radiofrequency card over a reader to trigger specific lighting effects and animations projected onto the walls and ceiling.

Furniture and Furnishings

Waiting areas and lobbies benefit from being furnished more like living rooms, with a variety of seating options to meet the comfort of the greatest number of persons. Integrated into the layout should be bariatric seating. No single chair will be comfortable for a person who may be tall or short, a pregnant woman, a person with a bad back, or someone who has just had a hip replacement. Having a variety of seating not only accommodates the widest range of persons but also has the benefit of looking more like a living room as opposed to an institutional waiting area.

Upholstery fabrics today have reached a high level of development in terms of durability and maintenance. Solution-dyed fibers will not fade in ultraviolet light, and they can be cleaned with a bleach solution. Many beautiful fabrics are available with Crypton backing, which has the comfort of a woven fabric on the outside with something akin to a vinyl coating on the back. In some situations, such as a high-back chair in a patient room, new vinyls with unusual color patterning and texture are very different from older vinyls that stuck to one's skin.

Interior Finishes

Interior finishes specifically developed for healthcare facilities enable designers to create esthetically beautiful environments without compromising infection control or ease of maintenance. It is important to remember that patients cannot evaluate the clinical competence of an institution, but they make a judgment nevertheless based on an assessment of the physical environment and their interactions with staff members. Visible attention to detail in the interior design of the setting generates feelings of confidence about the healthcare professionals who work there and the services provided.

In the past a highly waxed and buffed hard-surface floor evoked the desired image of cleanliness; indeed, many CEOs still find it difficult to get away from that idea. This is a mindset that hopefully will change. Manufacturers of hospital flooring have worked hard to develop products that do not need waxing. A life cycle study of flooring done by Florida Hospital determined that the "average cost to maintain the cheapest VCT [vinyl composition tile] floor over its lifetime is 9 to 15 times the initial cost of the floor . . . [whereas] the cost to maintain the most expensive floors like rubber and ceramic tile over their lifetime was less than the original installation cost of the floors" (Barnes 1998).

Carpet is the product of choice for nursing unit corridors for its ability to absorb sound and to cushion footsteps. In addition, it is gentle on the joints of aging nurses who are on their feet all day. Carpet is visually appealing to patients and associated with a hospitality ambience. Selecting the right carpet is essential. It should be designed for high-traffic healthcare settings and have permanent antimicrobial treatment and a moisture barrier.

Resistance to the use of carpet in nursing unit corridors is sometimes directed at infection control, but it need not be. Studies have shown that with hard-surface flooring particulates are kept airborne, whereas with carpet microorganisms are trapped until they are killed by antimicrobial treatments or removed by HEPA-(high-efficiency particulate air filter vacuum cleaners. With the proper carpet treatments, molds, mildew, fungi, and other microorganisms cannot multiply or cause odors.

Solution-dyed nylon fiber has the most permanent color, as the color is added at the time the fiber is extruded and stubborn stains can be cleaned with bleach. At one time solution-dyed fiber had limitations, but today it offers outstanding options. There are, however, other suitable nylon fibers that perform well in healthcare settings, such as type 6.6 DuPont Antron Legacy, BASF, and Solutia.

High-traffic corridors can be enhanced by a number of quality sheet-vinyl flooring products that have low-sheen finishes to reduce glare and falls. Esthetically, these products as a group are quite a departure from the institutional high-gloss floors often seen. They simulate a variety of natural materials such as stone or wood and require no wax.

It is increasingly common for patient rooms to have a wood-look vinyl floor. Such products are so realistic that it is difficult to tell it is not real wood, except that it performs better. For example, these floors may be antimicrobial, be antibacterial, be ntistatic, and require no waxing or buffing. Manufacturers are moving toward more environmentally friendly products made without chlorine or plasticizers, and considerable progress has been made for adhesives and backings with no off-gassing. Clearly, this is an important trend.

THE IMPORTANCE OF THE SERVICE SETTING

The environment delivers a message about the healthcare organization, its services, and quality long before the actual encounter takes place Fottler 2000). First impressions of the healthcare experience are often based on an evaluation of the physical environment and interactions with staff. As noted, patients can rarely assess the clinical care they are about to receive, but their confidence can be undermined or enhanced by their sensory perceptions of the setting.

Berry (2002) observes that patients are at a great knowledge disadvantage with the provider; to dispel fear they are especially attentive to what they can see and understand in the physical environment. Patients search for clues, each of which carries either a positive or negative message. The clues that comprise a customer experience are of two types: functional (did they fix the problem?) and emotional (smells, sounds, sights, textures, and the environment in which the service is offered) (Berry, Carbone, and Haeckel 2002). The built environment is a surrogate for the clinical experience.

What makes the healthcare service experience so unique is its intimacy—the consumer must be present to receive the service, which means that "The patient experiences what goes on in the service 'factory' and experiences the 'factory' itself" (Berry 2002). Upping the ante for patients in terms of anxiety, healthcare services are intangible, are technologically complex, and have high stakes. Add to that worries about medical errors, and one can agree with Berry's quip that "Being a patient is about the least amount of fun a consumer can buy. What is more stressful, frightening and emotionally draining than being a patient?"

Creating a Memorable Experience

Experiences can be designed, and more and more hospitals are paying attention to this to build market share, bond patients to their "brands," and simply meet their customers' expectations. Even the most generic of products, or in this case basic healthcare services such as drawing blood, are to the potential buyer what Levitt (1980) calls "a complex cluster of value satisfactions." Differentiation is not limited to giving the customer what is expected. What the customer expects may be augmented by things he never thought about. The augmented product or service is a condition of a mature market or relatively experienced or sophisticated customers (Levitt 1980).

The customer many are preparing for is that huge demographic— the baby boomers—that currently comprises 25 percent of the population, many of whom are approaching the age of 60. In the next 20 years they will require large amounts of healthcare services. Baby boomers are well-informed, are harder to please, and have greater expectations than any previous generation does. They expect convenience and comfort and are motivated by the power of choice. Remember, it was this group of women who, in their child-bearing years, demanded changes in the birthing experience that led to labor-delivery-recovery and labor-delivery-recovery-postpartum rooms; they refused to have their babies in operating rooms.

Imagine what changes members of this group will demand as they fill our healthcare facilities and how their expectations will cause them to shift their brand loyalty from one provider to another as they search for services packaged as a total experience. Conditioned by years of have-it-your-way retail marketing, baby boomers expect an array of amenity options offered in a healing environment setting by staff who are responsive, kind, and attentive.

Performing an Experience Audit

The process for performing an experience audit is discussed by Berry, Carbone, and Haeckel (2002) and illustrated by an example of a university hospital emergency department that undertook this task. The audit revealed minimal recognition of the emotional needs of patients and even less recognition for the needs of their families. In a careful analysis and documentation of the entire patient experience the task force created more than 100 positive experiential clues. These clues began with positioning signs saying "Hospital 3 Miles" to reassure people as they approached the facility, creating a less-confusing entrance for drive-up patients. The security guard became a greeter and roving ambassador, helping people navigate the registration process. The task force even improved the morgue experience. Overall, it eliminated many negatives that had previously never been noticed and added many emotionally positive clues.

Delivering the Brand

Patients are on a journey, whether it is to prevent disease and maintain wellness or to deal with a life-threatening illness. In either case they will have many encounters with your staff and ample opportunities to engage with the physical setting. Managing the evidence, or clues, associated with these experiences should not be left to chance. At Mayo Clinic, for example, "The patient comes first and this influences [everything from] the way it hires and trains employees, to the way it designs its facilities, to the way it approaches care. Mayo offers patients and their families concrete and convincing evidence of its strengths and values" (Berry and Bendapudi 2003).

If a hotel can keep a record of a customer's personal tastes in newspaper, music, and type of pillow, should not a hospital be able to make note of a few personal details that make the patient feel recognized and appreciated? Clearly, the life-altering events that occur in a hospital are often seared in our memories and have no equivalent in a hospitality setting. Nevertheless, healthcare organizations that systematically apply customer experience management principles will deliver a perception of value that engages consumer loyalty.

CONCLUSION

Both theory and research indicate that a well-designed setting can influence patient satisfaction, employee performance, and positive clinical outcomes. Fottler (2000) provides a thoughtful discussion of healing environments and a framework for action as well as the observation that "A healing environment is a holistic entity and not merely a set of separate components." It is as simple, and as complicated, as that.

REFERENCES

Barnes, S. R. 1998. "Life-Cycle Benefits of Flooring Surfaces in Health Care Applications." Florida Hospital, Unpublished report.

Berry, L. L. 2002. "Communicating Without Words." *Healthcare Design* (September): 15–18.

Berry, L. L., and N. Bendapudi. 2003. "Clueing in Customers." *Harvard Business Review* 81 (2): 2–7.

Berry, L. L., L. P. Carbone, and S. H. Haeckel. 2002. "Managing the Total Customer Experience." *MIT Sloan Management Review* 43 (3): 85–89.

Bower, G. 1981. "Mood and Memory." *American Psychologist* 36: 129–148.

Fottler, M. 2000. "Creating a Healing Environment: The Importance of the Service Setting in the New Consumer-Oriented Healthcare System." *Journal of Healthcare Management* 45 (2): 2.

Frampton, S. B., L. Gilpin, and P. A. Charmel. 2003. *Putting Patients First: Designing and Practicing Patient-Centered Care*. New York: Jossey-Bass.

Lemonick, M. 2005. "The Biology of Joy." *Time* (January) 17: A12–17.

Levitt, T. 1980. "Marketing Success Through Differentiation—of Anything." *Harvard Business Review* 58 (1): 83–91.

Linton, P. 1992. "Creating a Total Healing Environment." *Journal of Healthcare Design* 5 (1): 125–27.

Malkin, J. 1992. *Hospital Interior Architecture*. New York: John Wiley & Sons.

Niedenthal, P., M. Setterlund, and D. Jones. 1994. "Emotional Organization of Perceptual Memory." In *The Heart's Eye: Emotional Influences in Perception and Attention* edited by P. Niedenthal and S. Kitayana. Orlando, FL: Academic Press.

———. 2002. *Medical and Dental Space Planning: A Comprehensive Guide to Design, Equipment, and Clinical Procedures, 3rd Edition*. New York: John Wiley & Sons.

Pert, C. B. 1997. *Molecules of Emotion*. New York: Scribner.

Rabin, B. 1999. *Stress, Immune Function, and Health*. New York: Wiley-Liss.

Singer, J., and P. Salovey. 1988. "Mood and Memory: Evaluating the Network Theory Affect." *Clinical Psychology Review* 8: 211–51.

———. 2004. Keynote Speech. Presented at Healthcare Design conference, Houston, Texas, November 10.

Tennessen, C. M., and B. Cimprich. 1995. "Views to Nature: Effects on Attention." *Journal of Environmental Psychology* 15: 77–85.

Ulrich, R., and C. Zimring. 2004. *The Role of the Physical Environment in the Hospital of the 21st Century: A Once-in-a-lifetime Opportunity*. Concord, CA: The Center for Health Design.

CHAPTER 7

The Compelling Business Case for Better Buildings[1]

Blair Sadler, J.D., D. Kirk Hamilton, FAIA, FACHA;
Derek Parker, FAIA, RIBA, FACHA;
Leonard L. Berry, Ph.D.

> "We shape our buildings, and afterwards they shape us."
>
> —*Winston Churchill (1943)*

BUILDING A NEW facility is usually the biggest capital investment a CEO, medical staff, and board of trustees will ever make. Hospitals spent more than $17 billion on new construction in 2004, and in the years ahead spending on new hospital construction is expected to increase to $20 to $25 billion annually. With so much at stake, the time is right for hospital leaders to spend a little more money to build not just a new hospital but a better hospital, one that will actually save significant dollars in the long run.

When boards of trustees and organization leaders address the question of when and how to undertake a major facility expansion or replacement, they have traditionally considered five key issues:

1. **Urgency:** Is the expansion or replacement actually needed now to fulfill the mission, or can it be deferred? For example, are the market and volume assumptions sound, and have other external factors that would affect the decision been honestly and accurately considered?

2. **Appropriateness:** Is the proposed plan the most appropriate and sound? For example, have all alternatives been explored, such as partnerships with other hospitals and satellite operations as opposed to expanding or upgrading the facility in question?
3. **Cost:** Has the project been reviewed to offer the maximum value for every dollar spent? Is the cost appropriate for the expected level of construction quality?
4. **Financial impact:** Has the operating impact of the additional volume been accurately analyzed financially, and has the operating impact of not proceeding also been analyzed?
5. **Sources of funds:** Have the sources of funds for the new facility been identified? For example, is the combination of reserves, borrowing, philanthropy, and additional operating income reasonable and defensible?

All five questions must be addressed successfully for a board and CEO to responsibly proceed. All too often executives and their boards focus on the short-term issue of first cost when a careful review of long-term operating cost would better serve the organization's interests.

Today, there is a sixth, equally important question that must be addressed: has the project incorporated the new and emerging widely published literature on evidence-based building design's influence on the organization's business as well as the impact of quality, safety, and the built environment's on patients, families, and staff? The evidence is now so conclusive in many areas—and the financial impact so powerful—that it would be irresponsible for a board and CEO to proceed without fully including evidence-based design in their deliberations and decisions.

For example, based on the comprehensive research and conclusions described in chapters 3 and 4, there are several design innovations that every healthcare organization involved in a building project should implement without delay. These include but are not limited to (1) building larger single-bed rooms that reduce hospital-acquired (nosocomial) infections; (2) creating adaptable rooms by standard-izing shape, size, and headwalls, thus reducing unnecessary, costly, and dangerous patient transfers; (3) including double-door bath-room access to reduce patient falls and staff injuries; (4) installing hand-hygiene dispensers in each patient room to reduce staff-to-patient infections; (5) installing ceiling lifts and booms to reduce patient handling; and (6) providing positive distractions through art, restful views, and access to nature, thus relieving unnecessary stress and improving patient satisfaction.

THE STORY OF FABLE HOSPITAL

To fully understand the compelling business case for building bet-ter hospitals, based on published evidence and the experience of pio-neering organizations using evidence-based design to construct new facilities, we have created the hypothetical Fable Hospital. We chose to call our hospital Fable because it conveys the power of a story with a moral and evokes the nature of a legend. Although Fable Hospital does not yet exist, we believe several will be built in the next decade and that they will transform hospital design worldwide.

Fable Hospital is a new 300-bed regional medical center built to replace a 50-year-old facility that had 250 beds. Fable's per bed cost figure was $800,000. Located on a limited urban site, the hospital provides a comprehensive range of inpatient and ambulatory serv-ices, including medical and surgical, obstetrics, pediatrics, oncology, cardiac, and emergency. The cost of the total replacement project was $240 million.

Fable Hospital's core values include superior quality, safety, patient-focused care, family friendliness, staff support, cost sensitivity, envi-ronmental sustainability, and community responsibility. Management engaged a philosophically aligned design team based on the prem-ise that the building should reflect the organization's core values and strategic aspirations (Hamilton 2002). The designers responded with an array of design innovations and upgrades for the new facility, including the following:

- Oversized single rooms with dedicated space for patient, family, and staff activities and sufficient capacity for in-room procedures. The design maximizes daylight exposure to patient rooms and work spaces.
- Acuity-adaptable rooms standardized in shape, size, and headwall to eliminate the need to move patients as their condition changes.
- Double-door bathroom access to enable caregivers to more easily assist patients to and from the bathroom on foot or in wheelchairs.
- Decentralized, barrier-free nursing stations that place nurses in close proximity to their patients and supplies, most of which are stored in or near patient rooms.
- Alcohol-rub hand-hygiene dispensers located at the bedside in each patient room to reduce staff-to-patient transmission of pathogens.
- High-efficiency particulate air (HEPA) filters to improve the filtration of incoming outside air and eliminate recirculated air.
- Flexible spaces for advanced technologies, including operating rooms sized for robotic surgery, endovascular suites for minimally invasive surgery with sophisticated imaging, and imaging rooms designed to support continuous equipment advances.
- Peaceful settings, including artwork displays, space to listen to piano music, and gardens with fountains and benches, to moderate the stress of building occupants.
- Noise-reducing measures, including sound-absorbing floors and ceilings and a wireless communications system that eliminates overhead paging.
- Consultation spaces conveniently located to facilitate private communication between caregivers and families.
- Patient education centers on each floor offering brochures, books, videotapes, and access to the Internet.

- Internet access to disease-specific information and online support groups that improve patient and family understanding of illness.
- Staff support facilities, including a staff-only cafeteria, windowed break rooms with outside access, a day-care facility, and an exercise club.

These design innovations and upgrades collectively added $12 million to the construction budget, as shown in Table 7.1. In addition to these facility design investments, Fable invested in computerized order entry and bar code verification technology to minimize medication errors and to improve operational efficiency. The costs and benefits of these technology upgrades are not included in the tables in this chapter, which focus only on facility improvements. Combining the best of evidence-based design and the best of quality process improvements in hospitals will produce dramatic results.

Outcomes Measurement

Fable's CEO shared with the board an initial financial and performance impact assessment of the incremental facilities investment one year after occupying the new building. The assessment was based on management monitoring a series of key performance indicators in the 12 months since opening, part of a planned five-year evaluation program.

Seeking to be conservative in the analysis, the CEO adjusted downward certain estimates of increased savings and revenues to reflect positive influences other than the new building. The CEO wished to eliminate any concerns that the new facility was given more credit for improvements than warranted. The expense numbers also were adjusted to reflect the larger number of patients served in the new facility.

Even with the adjustments, the CEO was surprised by the significant first-year savings and revenue gains attributed to the facility. Table 7.2 shows the first-year financial gains the CEO presented

Table 7.1: Incremental Cost to Achieve a Better Building

Changes	Additional Cost	Calculations
Larger private patient rooms	$4,717,500	Based on an assumption of an increase of 100 square feet for each of 255 single patient rooms; 15 percent of the beds (45) are in an intensive care unit (ICU) configuration (100 sq. ft. x 255 rooms @ $185/sq. ft.)
Acuity-adaptable rooms	$816,000	Assumes additional medical gasses and monitor mounts in every room to provide ICU/stepdown capabilities with plug-in monitors (255 @ $3,200/room)
Larger windows	$150,000	The typical 3 ft. x 5 ft. patient room window is increased to 5 ft. x 8 ft. (300 @ $500/each)
Larger patient bathrooms with double-door access	$1,509,600	The larger space allows two staff members to assist a heavy patient to the toilet, and the enlarged doorway allows patient beds to be rolled in a sitting configuration closer to the bathroom (additional 32 sq. ft./toilet x 255 = 8,160 sq. ft. @ $185/sq. ft.)
Hand-hygiene facilities	$1,071,000	Hand-washing sink with foot pedals at the doorway to each acute patient room (alcohol-based hand-rub dispenser at the bedside: 255 @ $4,200/room)
Decentralized nursing substations	$556,800	Alcoves proximate to clusters of beds provide a charting surface, medication cassettes, supplies, alcohol-based hand-rub dispenser, and access to the information system (one per every four beds: 64 locations @ $8,700/unit)

Changes	Additional Cost	Calculations
Additional HEPA filters	$270,000	Installed HEPA 99.97% filtration on all air-handling units (AHUs) serving patient areas of the hospital (increases in motor horsepower and fan size of each AHU: 36 AHUs [25,000 CFM each] @ $7,500/unit)
Noise-reduction measures	$430,000	Construction materials were chosen for their sound absorption and control characteristics, and carpet was specified in most public areas. Upgraded ceiling and wall materials include additional layers of sheetrock for sound absorption and acoustical ceiling systems with higher noise-reduction efficiencies (upgrade for acoustical materials: $430,000)
Additional family and social spaces on each patient floor	$510,000	Added more public space in the form of a family-style great room and family kitchen on each patient floor (4 x 750 sq. ft, = 3,000 added sq. ft. @ $170/sq. ft.)
Health information resource center for patients and visitors	$95,200	Each patient floor has a resource center (4 x 140 sq. ft. = 560 sq. ft. @ $170/sq. ft.)
Meditation rooms on each floor	$61,200	Quiet spaces for family and staff meditation are located on each patient floor (4 x 90 sq. ft. = 360 sq. ft. x $170/sq. ft.)
Staff gym	$342,500	A gym with exercise machines, changing rooms, toilets, and showers is provided (1,500 sq. ft. @ $175/sq. ft. + allowance of $80,000 for equipment)

Changes	Additional Cost	Calculations
Art for public spaces and patient rooms	$450,000	Based on the assumption of an additional art allowance beyond the typical budget. Fable also rotates loaned artwork from local artists and solicits donated art (lighting enhancements to highlight selected artwork: $100,000; increase to art and sculpture allowance: $350,000)
Healing gardens (interior and exterior)	$1,050,000	Based on the assumption of additional sums above normal landscape cost for outdoor healing gardens, including a meditation garden, strolling garden, pond, outdoor meeting area, outdoor dining, and children's playground (increase to exterior landscape allowance: $900,000)
		The interior environment has been enhanced with indoor plantings, fountains, and atrium space (increase to interior design allowance: $150,000)
TOTAL	$12,029,800	

Note: All numbers are incremental increases above a typical hospital construction cost.

to the board and details how these numbers were derived. The table indicates that after one year the incremental costs are virtually recovered and that significant financial benefit will then accrue year after year. In all cases the numbers presented in Table 7.2 are based on performance results of organizations participating in The Center for Health Design's Pebble Project research initiative—that is, they are based on actual results.

Table 7.2: Financial Impact of Design Decisions

Evidence	Savings	Calculations
Patient Falls: Reduced	$2,452,800	Patient falls are common and can cause significant harm. Falls result from patient instability, confusion, unfamiliar surroundings, lack of assistance, poor lighting, and slippery surfaces.

The national unlitigated average cost of a fall is $10,000 (Hendrich 1995); litigated falls can cost millions of dollars. Like many other hospitals, Fable is self-insured because of the high cost of malpractice insurance. The cost of patient falls goes directly to the bottom line.

The national median rate of acute care falls is 3.5 falls/1,000 patient days; this was the rate experienced by Fable's predecessor hospital. Fable reduced patient falls by 80% by locating toilets closer to the patient, putting double doors in bathrooms, utilizing bed exit features that notify a nurse when a patient is out of bed, decentralizing nursing stations, and locating supplies close by to reduce the amount of time the nurse is away from the patient. Fable's reduced patient falls rate is the same as that experienced by Pebble partner Clarian Health Partners Methodist Hospital in Indianapolis, Indiana (Flynn 2003; Hendrich, Bender, and Nyhuis 2003).

(Savings: 300 beds at 80% occupancy = 240 beds = 87,600 patient days/1,000 x 3.5 = 306 falls/year x $10,000 = $3,066,000; falls reduced by 80% = savings of $2,452,800[1])

Table 7.2: *(continued)*

Evidence	Savings	Calculations
Patient transfers: Reduced	$3,893,200	Transferring patients to a different room creates additional direct and indirect costs. Transfers increase the risk of medication errors and patient falls, add nursing time for transporting and assessing patients, require extra transport equipment, and contribute to hospital flow inefficiencies. Multiple transfers reduce the continuity of patient care as more caregivers become involved in the care process. Including only the direct costs of additional nursing labor, laundry and linen, and equipment usage, the estimated average cost of one patient room transfer is $250 to $300 (Hendrich and Lee 2003). It is not uncommon for hospital patients to be moved three or four times. The facility that Fable replaced averaged one transfer per patient. Because of its acuity-adaptable rooms, Fable reduced patient transfers by 80%. Fable's experience is consistent with that of Clarian Health Partners Methodist Hospital, which reduced patient transfers by 90% in its redesigned, acuity-adaptable cardiac critical care unit (Hendrich, Fay, and Sorrells 2004). (Savings: 19,466 patient stays x $250 = $4,866,500 x 80% = $3,893,200)
Nosocomial infections: Reduced	$80,640	Recent estimates in the literature of the incidence of nosocomial infections in hospitals range from about 5% of patients (Gardner 2002) to nearly 10% of patients (Burke 2003). Infections are more

Table 7.2: *(continued)*

Evidence	Savings	Calculations
		likely in multi-bed rooms because of the cross-transmission of microbial pathogens between patients.
		The average cost of additional hospitalized treatment associated with nosocomial infections was estimated in one report to be in excess of $7,000 (in 1985 dollars) (Burrington 1999). Pebble partner Bronson Methodist Hospital in Kalamazoo, Michigan, estimates that each nosocomial infection averages $4,000 in additional costs; Bronson is reimbursed for 58% of these additional costs.
		Fable reduced its nosocomial infection rate by four patients per month by having 100% single rooms, HEPA filters, and increased hand hygiene stations. Like Bronson, 58% of added infection-related costs were reimbursed.
		Bronson reduced infections in four to six patients a month after occupying its new facility (Sandrick 2002). Bronson has 287 staffed beds.
		(Savings: 4/month at $4,000 unlitigated cost = $192,000/year x 42% = $80,640)
Drug costs: Reduced	$1,216,666	Drugs are an inevitable and expensive part of hospitalization, averaging 14.9%, or $2,448, of the overall average cost per stay of $16,438 in 2000 (Solucient 2002).
		Fable carefully measured pre- and postoccupancy drug usage based on the literature, drawing a connection between

Table 7.2: *(continued)*

Evidence	Savings	Calculations
		positive distractions in the environment (e.g., art, music, landscape, family involvement) and patients' reduced need for pain medication (Rubin, Owens, and Golden 1998).
		Fable reduced overall per patient pain medication use by 5%, a result supported by a 16% drop in medication use reported for Pebble partner Karmanos Hospital in Detroit, Michigan, for sickle-cell patients using redesigned facilities (Shepard and Mersch 2001). Fifty percent of Fable's reduced drug costs were savings; the other 50% were reimbursed.
		(Savings: 87,600 patient days/4.5 days = 19,466 patient stays x $2,500/stay x 5% = $2,433.333/2 = $1,216,666)
Nursing turnover: Reduced	$164,000	The healthcare industry is suffering a severe skilled labor shortage that includes nurses. High rates of skilled labor turnover plague the industry. Because of the emotional and physical stress of healthcare work and its long hours, the design of the facility plays a particularly important role in staff attraction and retention.
		The national full-time equivalent (FTE) per occupied bed average is 5.45 staff (Ingenix 2003). Fable's staff equals 1,308 FTEs, of whom 30%, or 391, are nurses. The overall appeal of Fable's facility and specific staff amenities such as break, daycare, and exercise facilities contributed to Fable reducing nurse turnover

Evidence	Savings	Calculations
		from 14% to 10%. These data track the reduced turnover of nurses at Bronson Methodist Hospital after occupying its new building.
		The estimated cost of one nurse turnover varies widely in the literature (The HSM Group 2002). One report estimates the average cost for recruitment, orientation, and retention of a critical care nurse to be $64,000 ("Two Hospitals . . ." 2002). Fable estimates its cost to replace one nurse is $20,500. This figure is derived from recruitment costs, higher registry nursing costs during recruitment, and orientation costs. Fable attributes 50% of the credit for its reduced nursing turnover to the new facility and the other 50% to salary adjustments and other retention initiatives.
		(Savings: 39 nurses leaving [10% of 391] instead of 55 nurses [14%] = $328,000 saved [$20,500/turnover]/2 = $164,000)
	Increased Revenue	
Market share: Increased	$2,168,100	Fable increased its market share by 1.5%. Fable's increase is consistent with Bronson Methodist Hospital, which increased its market share by more than 2% in 2001 and 2002, its first two post-occupancy years.
		Fable's market share gain boosted net patient days by 1,314; its net patient revenue per diem is $2,200, a figure consistent with Bronson's performance

Table 7.2: *(continued)*

Evidence	Savings	Calculations
		in its new facility. To be conservative Fable attributes 75% of its market share gain to the new facility.
		(Net revenue: 1,314 additional patient days x $2,200 = $2,890,800 x 75% = $2,168,100)
Philanthropy: Increased	$1,500,000	Fable's new facility played an important role in increasing philanthropic contributions from about $5 million a year before construction of the new building to $6.5 million during the first year of occupancy. Naming opportunities in the new facility encouraged increased giving, as did the building's tangible representation of Fable's vision for healthcare in the community.
		Fable's increased contributions are consistent with the experience of Pebble partner Children's Hospital and Health Center in San Diego, California. Management believes the impact of its innovatively designed Rose Pavilion Building was instrumental in raising $5 million during and immediately following construction.
TOTAL	$11,475,406[2]	

Notes:
1 In the interest of conservatism we have assumed all of Fable's acute care patient falls to be unlitigated; in actuality, some of these falls would be litigated and Fable's costs would be significantly higher in these cases. Thus, Fable's estimated savings resulting from reducing patient falls by 80% are understated by the exclusion of litigation-related costs from our calculations.

2 This figure, representing the estimated total reduced costs and increased revenues for Fable Hospital's first year of operation in its new facility, is on the low side. First, we sought to be conservative in all estimates to strengthen the

credibility of our message. Given that Fable Hospital is built from the experiences of multiple hospitals and research streams, we wished to err on the side of under- rather than overpromising. Second, Fable is benefiting in ways not reflected in the table because of insufficient data available to credibly present hard numbers that can be attributed to facility design innovation. Reduced medication errors aided by design features such as better lighting and less noise (in addition to the process improvements of bar coding and computerized order entry) is an example.

A Reality Check

Is Fable Hospital a pipedream? Can a more expensive building that is better for patients and their caregivers actually provide the financial gains shown in the Fable case study? With values-driven hospital leadership, supportive hospital boards, talented designers, and a willingness to embrace the lessons of evidence-based design, the answer is, "Yes."

GETTING STARTED

A healthcare executive or trustee who wishes to follow a path similar to Fable Hospital might ask, "How best to begin?" The path begins with the vision that positive impacts on patients, staff, and the community will occur through a collaborative commitment to combining the best design evidence with the core values and belief systems of the organization. Thus, a first step is to formally define and widely disseminate this vision and keep it in front of organizational members at all times.

The second step is to become familiar with the work of the pathfinders who are blazing the trail for others. This can include reading, attending conferences, and taking benchmarking tours of exemplary projects. One wise measure would be to ensure that the organization's guiding coalition grasps the importance of an evidence-based course for decision making on design and construction projects. Another would be to assemble a strong collaborative team of advisors who have the complementary skills and experience to rigorously follow such a course. A team of programming consultants, architects, engineers, and interior designers who value evidence-based design might be bolstered with social scientists such as an environmental psychologist or an expert in performance improvement (Hamilton 2003). The prudent executive should be prepared to invest extra time preparing a sophisticated description of the project that goes beyond a simple listing of proposed space requirements. It is helpful to be able to describe a project's goals and objectives with clarity, including hypotheses concerning outcomes expected from the design.

Resistance to a process that differs from prevailing practice can come from almost any source. In addition to the predictable resistance to any form of change, the team can expect to be challenged at first by skeptics who will question the evidence, financial assumptions, and link between facility design and clinical outcomes. This is why a certain amount of study and a team accustomed to rigor will be useful. The challenge to financial assumptions will require careful analysis and cautious budgeting that avoids overreliance on previous budget or cost models. It would be wise to involve the external consultants early in the process to gain the maximum benefit from their experience.

A typical barrier to success is expecting a project to neatly fit into the same budget and schedule as a conventional project, when in fact it likely will require an extended predesign phase to properly define the scope; identify, analyze, prioritize, and integrate design innovations; and plan an assessment protocol. The team should be prepared to do more sophisticated life cycle costing than occurs in a conventional project, as fewer decisions will be based exclusively on the lowest first cost. Just as engineers might recommend a more expensive air-conditioning system because of its superior energy performance over the project's life cycle, the ongoing operational costs of alternate designs should be compared before a design is selected. A savvy executive will insist on using multiple before-and-after measures to assess the project, including financial, clinical, and satisfaction indicators.

THE MORAL OF THE STORY

Illness costs—both human suffering and financial expenditures—exact high prices. Conversely, well-being pays dividends—both persons and profits are healthier. Investment in better healthcare buildings pays off directly and indirectly through enhanced patient care and employee well-being.

In a world that has begun to understand its resources as finite, maximizing the benefits realized for every dollar invested becomes crucial. The business case for better hospital buildings is strong. In this composite case study of Fable Hospital, based on the actual performance of Pebble Project facilities, our estimated savings and revenue gains nearly recapture the incremental investment in a better building in just the first year despite a deliberate effort to be conservative.

Fable Hospital does not exist on one site or in one facility, but it is not an invention either. Benefits associated with its design innovations are actually being achieved. Fable serves as an idealized template to demonstrate how evidence-based design can improve patient and staff satisfaction, medical outcomes, safety, cost efficiency, resource conservation, and financial performance. In sharing the Fable concept with several audiences in the United States and Europe, we have seen considerable interest in the concept.

CONCLUSION

Most hospital boards or management leaders have only one or two opportunities in their professional lives to create a permanent legacy that will transform their organization and community through designing and building an optimal healing facility. It is an opportunity that should not be wasted.

Typically, boards and CEOs address five key issues when considering whether and how to undertake a major facility expansion or replacement: (1) urgency, (2) appropriateness, (3) cost, (4) financial impact, and (5) sources of funds. It is now essential that they include a sixth issue: whether the project incorporated the relevant literature on evidence-based building design and its relevance to the business, quality, and safety impact on patients, families, and staff.

We believe that the lesson for all healthcare organizations is clear: provide a built environment that is welcoming to patients, improves their quality of life, and supports families and employees, or suffer the economic consequence in a competitive environment. As healthcare leaders, we have an extraordinary opportunity and serious responsibility to truly build better hospitals—hospitals that actually facilitate physical, mental, and social well-being and productive behavior in their occupants. In addition, through measured superior performance we can actually improve our organizations' financial results over the long term.

NOTE

1. This chapter was adapted with permission from Berry et al. (2004).

REFERENCES

Berry, L. L., D. Parker, R. Coile, D. K. Hamilton, D. O'Neill, and B. Sadler. 2004. "Can Better Buildings Improve Care and Increase Your Financial Returns?" *Frontiers of Health Services Management* 21 (1): 3–24.

Burke, J. 2003. "Patient Safety: Infection Control—A Problem for Patient Safety." *New England Journal of Medicine* 348: 651–56.

Burrington, M. 1999. *Can Private Rooms Be Justified in Today's Healthcare Market?* Houston, TX: Center for Innovation in Health Facilities.

Children's Hospital Today. 2002. "Two Hospitals, One Goal: Retaining PICU Nurses." [Online article; retrieved 08/22/05.] www.childrenshospitals.net.

Churchill, W. 1943. "Famous Quotes and Stories of Winston Churchill." [Online information; retrieved 5/15/05.] http://www.winstonchurchill.org.

Flynn, L. 2003. "Matters of the Heart." *Building Design & Construction* (February): 38–44, 57.

Gardner, M. 2002. "Aseptic Technique Is in Your Hands." *Infection Control Today.* 6 (5): 22.

Hamilton, D. K. 2002. "First Design the Organization, then Design the Building!" *Interiors & Sources* (January/February): 94–95.

———. 2003. "The Four Levels of Evidence-based Practice." *Healthcare Design* (November), 18–26.

Hendrich, A. L. 1995. *Falls, Immobility, and Restraints: A Resource Manual.* Philadelphia, PA: CV Mosby.

Hendrich, A. L., J. Fay, and A. Sorrells. 2004. "Effects of Acuity-Adaptable Rooms on Flow of Patients and Delivery of Care." *American Journal of Critical Care.* 13 (1): 35–45.

—————. Forthcoming. "Cardiac Comprehensive Critical Care: The Impact of Acuity-Adaptable Patient Rooms on Current Patient Flow Bottlenecks and Future Care Delivery." *American Journal of Critical Care.*

Hendrich, A. L., P. S. Bender, and A. Nyhuis. 2003. "Validation of the Hendrich's II Falls Risk Model: A Large Concurrent Case/Control Study of Hospitalized Patients." *Applied Nursing Research* 16 (1): 9–21.

Hendrich, A. L., and N. Lee. 2003. "Intra-Unit Hospital Patient Transfers: A Time and Motion Cost Analysis Study." Working paper.

The HSM Group. 2002. "Acute Care Hospital Survey of R.N. Vacancy and Turnover Rates in 2000, 9." Chicago: American Organization of Nurse Executives.

Ingenix. 2003. *The 2003 Almanac of Hospital Financial & Operating Indicators: A Comprehensive Benchmark of the Nation's Hospitals.* Salt Lake City, UT: Ingenix.

Rubin, H. R., A. J. Owens, and G. Golden. 1998. *An Investigation to Determine Whether the Built Environment Affects Patients' Medical Outcomes.* Concord, CA: The Center for Health Design.

Sandrick, K. 2002. "Designing a Defense." *Health Facilities Management* May, 14–19.

Shepard, D., and G. Mersch. 2001. "Creation of a Healing Environment in a Clinical Cancer Center." In *Proceedings of the 26th Annual Oncology Nursing Society Congress.* Pittsburgh, PA: Oncology Nursing Society.

Solucient, LLC. 2002. *The DRG Handbook: Comparative Clinical and Financial Benchmarks.* Evanston, IL: Solucient, LLC.

CHAPTER 8

Cultural Transformation and Design

D. Kirk Hamilton, FAIA, FACHA, and Robin Diane Orr, M.P.H.

THE CASE FOR profound change in healthcare is strong. Costs are soaring, infection rates and errors are at unacceptable levels, patients are not satisfied, nurses are leaving the profession, doctors are feeling powerless, the aging infrastructure of hospitals funded by Hill-Burton legislation is increasingly obsolete, and information technology is lagging far behind that of other industries. While there is a sense that the system itself is broken, there is no consensus or widespread commitment on how to repair or replace it.

To effect profound change in healthcare we must look deeply into the very soul of our organizations to inspire the hearts and minds of those working at the bedside, in admitting, housekeeping, and administrative offices. It is their passion and talents that need to be unleashed to create the hospital of the future. We need to create cultures in healthcare organizations that are uplifting, inspiring, and supportive of the human spirit. Successful organizational cultures that have survived and thrived over time find a way to acknowledge that the work of everyone is meaningful. It is not by accident that such cultures flourish. Our challenge is to not only design buildings based on evidence but to design the culture that will thrive instead of merely survive in these buildings. We desperately need to redesign our organizations to rekindle a commitment to healing, hope, optimism, innovation, and creativity.

CULTURE AS RELATED TO FACILITIES, ENVIRONMENT, AND PERFORMANCE

It is unlikely that profound change can be accomplished without a simultaneous effort to dramatically alter both the culture and facilities of an organization. Leaders who identify gaps between the character of a desired organization and the current reality need to have the courage to change the organization's course and steer for an improved future. Important behavioral change is unlikely without a positive change in organizational culture. The physical environment can powerfully support the desired behaviors or discourage undesirable actions. Thus, facility design becomes an important tool for executives planning cultural change.

Culture is sometimes described as "the way we do things around here." The organization's culture is a powerful set of norms, habits, policies, and procedures that guide behavior. The artifacts and outward signs of the culture are based on the organization's values— both expressed and observed—along with deep underlying assumptions (Schein 1992). The physical environment is a pervasive and ever-present artifact of the organization's culture. The environment continuously offers cultural clues to members of the organization and all who come into contact with it. The organization's environment—and therefore its design—can be a crucial enabler of desired behaviors, or it can be a barrier to the desired behavior and play a powerful role in preventing the intended culture.

The symbols of culture appear from the moment one encounters the site and include signage, landscape or urban context, layout of the property, drives, parking, plantings, and site amenities. The design of a campus and appearance of each building can be attractive and welcoming, ambiguous and confusing, or simply forbidding. Some hospitals have parking lots that could have been designed for a discount store, whereas others have parking areas with trees, flowers, and soothing music. These nonverbal cues signal something about the organization and make an important first impression.

There are obvious differences between healthcare organizations whose buildings feature soaring lobbies full of plaques recognizing prominent donors, those whose pleasantly lit lobbies are filled with friendly welcoming faces, and those whose dim and dusty lobbies are simply vestibules leading to a bleak set of confusing corridors. The space in which patients are met and the actions of those they encounter begin to tell those patients how they will be perceived and how the organization might care for them. These silent signals sent by the building are everywhere we look, including the patient's room. Surely the stay and expectations of its outcomes can be very different when the room is pleasant, is cheery, and encourages visitors rather than when the room is dismal, cold, and foreboding.

There is, of course, no single culture that would suit every hospital or healthcare organization. Each organization has its own unique culture forged from the distinctive combination of circumstance, leadership, and evolution. An infinite number of cultures are possible in a healthcare organization. Figure 8.1 offers a few generic, high-level examples.

Is one culture better than another? The ideal culture is individually suited to the specific organization and unique economic, social,

---

Figure 8.1: Broad Cultural Roles Healthcare Organizations Might Adopt

Science and learning	Patient centered
Safety	Family centered
Strive for excellence	Planetree
Competence	Religious sponsor
Efficiency	Catholic culture of caring
Research and teaching	Eden alternative
"We know you here"	Bottom-line business
Independent practice	Investor owned
Community service	Urban vitality
Carriage trade	Small-town character
Blue collar	Magnet nursing
Indigent or charity	Technology focus
Military	Narrow specialization
Children's	Surgery

---

and political context in which the organization finds itself. In some cases two different labels for culture may exist in the same organization. If a hospital is especially committed to improving patient safety, for instance, that goal can be achieved through cultures of safety, excellence, or clinical quality. A culture of caring for individuals may appear at a faith-based organization or a community-based institution. No particular culture is superior for all institutions, but each individual organizational situation must have a unique culture. Thus, it is important for organizations to work at building their own individualized and effective cultures and develop an ideal fit for their purposes.

The roots of culture run deep, based on unspoken but closely held beliefs and powerful basic assumptions. This is one reason culture is so difficult to change. Many attempts at cultural change fail as the power of the preexisting culture overcomes the change initiative and behavior snaps back to the prior state. Successful cultural change initiatives require focused investment of time and energy until the foundation of shared assumptions shifts enough to support the new culture. Permanently establishing a major change in the culture of a healthcare organization probably takes between three and seven years (Andrews et al. 1994).

The tendency for culture to persist in the face of a change initiative is one of the reasons a simultaneous change in facility design is recommended. As mentioned, a well-designed physical environment can be both a barrier to undesired behaviors and an enabler of desired behavior. The current physical environment in some way probably supports the existing culture. If change is desired, the physical environment can encourage new behaviors, which then lead to a fresh new image and positive operational outcomes. The setting can be changed to discourage the old paradigm and support the new image, work processes, and intended behaviors.

CULTURAL CHANGE AND IMPROVEMENT

There are many examples and rays of hope in the quest for more effective healthcare delivery models. The pioneers who founded Planetree raised awareness of the critical need for a more patient-

and consumer-centered approach. More than 60 organizations have adopted some or all of Planetree's innovative philosophy. Planetree's Mid-Columbia Medical Center in The Dalles, Oregon, was an early example of hospitalwide cultural change blended with a facility makeover. The Planetree headquarters in Derby, Connecticut, is a more recent example. Hospitals in the United States, and many around the world, have been influenced to some degree by Planetree's passionate case for greater attention to the needs of patients and their families. (See Chapter 6 for further discussion of the Planetree model.) The actual experience at such organizations extends beyond the positive impact on patient satisfaction. Individuals who work in organizations imbued with these values find great meaning in their work, affecting outcomes on several levels.

An early example of physical change affecting behavior was demonstrated at a Planetree model unit, Trinity Medical Center in Moline, Illinois. Step one was to demolish the old nursing station and replace it with a new one. The original was a fortress for nurses, who sat behind a glass wall, enclosed in an industrially manufactured booth. They communicated through a window located in a forbidding hallway of hard surfaces and glaring fluorescent light. Staff behavior and patient and family behavior were predictable. Staff would virtually ignore family members as if they were intruding into their territory. Family member would feel as if they were not welcome and interaction with staff was off limits.

Step two was to replace the imposing nursing station with an open wooden desktop spilling into a carpeted space with indirect lighting, comfortable guest chairs, and an aquarium. The area features a round table and chairs for family conferences. The result was that behaviors did change. The more open setting encouraged interactions among families and staff. Families felt more comfortable and thus less anxious in stressful situations; in fact, it was impossible to sustain the prior behaviors in the new environment. In this case the design of the physical environment prohibited a return to the former, undesired culture. When physical barriers are designed into a facility it creates a "we" versus "them" mentality. Communication in the previous culture was restricted. Patients and their families felt alienated and closed out, and in some cases even as if they were in the way. The cold, harsh environment perpetuated a culture that was dehumanizing and diminished the opportunity for quiet, comfortable, direct interactions.

What comes first, the chicken or the egg? Cultural change or facility change? At Parrish Medical Center in Titusville, Florida, CEO George Mikitarian began a cultural change effort after the organization's replacement building was in place and new patterns and behaviors seemed desirable. At Mid-Columbia Medical Center, CEO Mark Scott made a commitment to adopt the Planetree philosophy of patient-centered care and invested in a major cultural change before renovating the building in a way designed to support the new model.

Although either sequence can produce positive results, one study has shown that a simultaneous effort that combines design of a new culture with design of new facilities offers synergy and increases effectiveness (Hamilton 2003). Barney Johnson, CEO of Harbor Hospital in Baltimore, led an effort to design the organization's new culture and physical environment jointly. It is clear that changes to the physical environment made possible some of the changes in work processes and symbolized Harbor's commitment to profound change. The result of a combined cultural and facility change was a well-documented, dramatic turnaround in terms of finances and stakeholder satisfaction (Copeland, Johnson, and Orr 1997).

An Integrated Model for Transformational Change

The greatest impact of positive change is being achieved by those who understand the issue as one of a whole system and act in a broad manner. They simultaneously implement system and process redesign with facility redesign and cultural change initiatives. This is not easy, and perhaps because it is not, few healthcare managers are using all the tools at their disposal to effect positive change in their organizations.

There has also been an unfortunate disconnect between the physical design of healthcare facilities and the development of outcomes at the operational, clinical, and service levels. Architects are able to design buildings that include many features that can contribute to creation of a healing environment, but they are unable to change culture, operational model, or staff attitudes. Behaviors that do not support the design's intent can diminish the effectiveness of the facility's impact. At the same time, well-meaning individuals can implement initiatives intended to shift an organization's culture, but all too often efforts including independent and unconnected activities, fail as behaviors return to "the way we do things around here."

Organizational theory supports the concept of simultaneous interventions to generate change. Sociotechnical theory (Appelbaum 1997) suggests that joint optimization of the social aspects (including culture) and technical aspects (including architecture) of an organization will more often deliver the desired results. This strongly suggests that healthcare executives leading a change process should work simultaneously with both organizational consultants and architects who actively collaborate. It also suggests that architects and organizational consultants should more often integrate their activities.

A Strong Leader Points the Way

An initiative aimed at transformational change has no chance for success without the total genuine support of the top leadership. Culture is one of the important responsibilities of leadership. Leaders interested in pointing the way to positive, transformational change in their organizations must convene a forum to discuss and plan for change. The ideal forum for designing the desired culture and planning the interventions needed to achieve it should include an interdisciplinary group with broad representation and a number of potential energized champions. Make sure those who work at all levels are fully involved. Consider active representation of patients and members of the community. Consider involving your consultants from the beginning, as an outsider's view of your organization is essential and may encourage you to cross traditional boundaries. This is not a time for silo thinking or silo processes.

CHARTING A COURSE FOR CHANGE

Just as the architects and engineers will conduct a facility assessment, so must the organization and its consultants perform a cultural assessment. Such an assessment explores the stated and observed cultures as well as underlying perceptions of the organization's members. An assessment addresses an organization's customs, symbols, policies, procedures, attitudes, behaviors, expectations, norms, stated and underlying values, and aspects of the environment that contribute to culture (Mallak et al. 2003a). One type of assessment focuses on observations of behavior and critical incidents (Mallak et al. 2003b).

To chart a course to a new place you must know where to begin and the intended destination. Architects might assist in preparing a vision and goal statement to guide the design for new facilities. Similarly, an organizational consultant should work with the leadership to define the desired culture. The gap between the culture discovered in the assessment and the culture desired by the vision is the subject of potential interventions that can be designed to close it.

Take an appreciative look at the best things your organization is doing and build on your strengths. Find ways to celebrate and increase the best you have to offer. Empower the change team to embrace discovery, take risks, and challenge the status quo (Christensen, Bohmer, and Kenagy 2000).

Benchmarking successful healthcare organizations can be useful but may not be the "right" or only answer for your organization. What are others doing? Aggressively adopt and refine good ideas. Ensure that examples from outside the healthcare world are explored. A well-run airline may offer lessons in arrival and departure or automated registration. A shipping company may help you understand your supply chain. A gourmet coffee shop may teach you about customer appeal and service. A retail setting may offer lessons about convenient access and parking.

A successful effort to create transformational change must address many aspects of an organization. Examine your leadership actions and behavior for unintended signals. Inventory your organization's best practices to create a culture of learning and sharing. Review your orientation process, education, training, staff development, and mentorship programs. What language do you use to describe your organization? What is the first impression for a new hire? Examine the organization itself. Does the organizational structure illustrated on a chart provide an effective model for performance and communication, or do people routinely operate outside the official structure to get things done? How do you measure performance? What do you do with the feedback from measurement?

Plan the Change Process

The range of choices for planned interventions is broad and includes leadership initiatives, team-building workshops, interpersonal and group process interventions, organizational process initiatives, work design efforts, reengineering, technology applications, organizational restructuring, revisions to policies and procedures, empowerment initiatives, performance measurement, quality initiatives, service training, customer relations management, orientation and mentorship initiatives, staff development interventions, strategic planning, and cultural change efforts. Do not forget the vital importance of potential facility changes in support of your other efforts.

The combination of interventions best suited to your organization must be planned together and their implementation must be integrated to obtain the best results. No single intervention is sufficient to turn the powerful inertia of an entrenched culture in a new direction. Piecemeal efforts will undermine your ultimate goal. The various interventions and change initiatives should result in complete alignment among the organization's stated goals, its strategy, the organizational structure and processes to achieve it, the positive and uplifting culture, as well as the appropriate facilities and technology to effectively support the ongoing complex activity.

Organizations planning a patient- and family-centered culture might institute several programs such as an initiative to provide greater patient education and complete access to medical information. Such an organization would undertake an effort to create a healing environment, using evidence-based design to alter the character of its healthcare setting. The organization would examine its place within the continuum of care and healing, developing initiatives to extend its influence upstream and downstream into the system. For example, special attention might be paid to ethical considerations in the final stages of life. Consideration could be given to new partners and relationships in the healing arts and the offering of complementary therapies. This might include an extensive massage therapy program supporting both patients and staff. Music therapy, performing arts, humor programs, pet therapy, and art therapy might be implemented. An organization moving in this direction would likely work carefully to develop customer service standards and fully understand and improve aspects of the patient's experience.

The combination of interventions at another organization might be very different. John Reiling, CEO of St. Joseph's Community Hospital in West Bend, Wisconsin, is passionately focused on creating a culture of safety. St. Joseph's initiatives included convening a learning lab of experts to share safety concepts from high-reliability organizations such as NASA, the airlines, and nuclear industries (Center for the Study of Healthcare Management 2002). The organization used failure mode analysis to evaluate all of its own work processes. The resulting facility design uses precise standardization and repetitive design to eliminate confusion.

Integrated Implementation of Change

Implementation of change initiatives can be complex. There may be many overlapping and mutually supporting initiatives, often with different leaders and champions. They may begin and end at different dates and times, involving different constituencies. The pace of change may be slow and the results difficult to measure.

Every decision you make is a single brick in the new structure you are creating. Make sure these decisions are pointing the organization in the intended direction. Every meeting, memo, policy, and decision should be evaluated through the lens of the cultural and philosophical model. Check yourself continuously for consistency of message. You will discover an endless number of large and small teachable moments, all of which must be recognized and leveraged to full advantage. Retreats for staff and physicians are an effective way to keep attention on the change issue and signal management's commitment. Getting away from the day-to-day situation can help focus attention on the desired culture. Think of your education and training efforts as a crucial investment in the engagement of your employees. Education and training should be seen as a process, not an event.

Embarking on a cultural transformation process (see Figure 8.2) will require finding fresh new ways to communicate a heartfelt message that inspires, educates, and informs all stakeholders. You will need to develop measures to gauge your progress on this long journey as well as a simple dashboard of these indicators to give you frequent feedback as you steer the new course. Measurement must be a serious commitment of leadership. If you are not measuring the important things, you can easily miss your target.

The Journey Does Not End

The process does not stop when the change has been accomplished. Sustaining successful change comprises a completely different set of tasks and ongoing commitment. Vigilance is required to support the new change because culture is so persistent and will tend to reassert itself long after the desired change has been implemented. This attention means an effort to assess culture at intervals, continuing to promote and reinforce the new culture through orientation, refresher courses, mentorship, and rewards and recognition—a few of the many potential ongoing techniques to firmly embed the new model.

CONCLUSION

Profound change of the U.S. healthcare delivery system and dramatic improvement at every individual healthcare organization are sorely needed. The most powerful way to implement transforma-

Figure 8.2: Cultural Transformation Checklist

Start at the Top	✓
1. The CEO must make a personal and organizational commitment to embark on a journey of cultural transformation.	
2. This is not the "program of the month."	
3. Make a long-term commitment to the transformation process.	
4. Make it become "the way we do things around here."	

Get Your Leadership on Board	✓
1. Leadership at every level understands why you are embarking on cultural transformation.	
2. Make a commitment to support or get out of the way.	
3. Be visible and caring.	

Convey a Message that Is Compelling and Urgent	✓
1. Relay it in language that is consistent with your existing mission and values and your new visionary language, which is compelling and able to galvanize the heads and hearts of your organization.	

Select Champions	✓
1. Convene a design team that will lead the transformation process.	
2. Have monthly meetings to share progress, eliminate barriers, and move forward.	
3. Hardwire changes into the fabric of your organization.	

Integrate Facility Design with Culture Design	✓
1. Configure the facility to support the culture.	
2. Have your design team collaborate and partner with the culture design team.	
3. Make sure that all architectural design decisions support desired behaviors and performance outcomes.	
4. Make sure the design team you select is knowledgeable about and will be an advocate for the cultural transformation process.	

Listen, Communicate, and Learn	✓
1. Build on the positive.	
2. Have your finger on the pulse of the organization.	
3. Learn from the best in your organization, the healthcare industry, and outsiders.	

Tie to Performance	✓
1. Have a strong bias toward action.	
2. Remember that what gets measured gets done.	
3. Do not get hung up on traditional metrics.	
4. Letters from patients and staff are useful feedback to validate that you are on the right path.	

Celebrate Wins	✓
1. Every action that builds on your culture is a transformational step.	
2. Remember to have fun.	
3. You are on the wrong path if it is not a journey of innovation, creativity, and personal achievement.	

tional change is through an integrated process in which culture, work process, and facility design can be addressed simultaneously with the intention to achieve joint optimization.

Visionary leaders must point the way to a better future, launch the change process, protect the champions, nourish their efforts, and celebrate the successes every day. Such a process demands an interdisciplinary team committed to synergistic collaboration and prepared to passionately devote long hours over several years to achieve the goal. Many champions are needed to play many important roles. Most of all, there must be a commitment to act.

To foster profound and positive change is noble work in the cause of all who come into contact with these organizations. It is work that must begin and continue at most of our hospitals, medical centers, and healthcare systems.

REFERENCES

Andrews, H., L. Cook, J. Davidson, D. Schurman, E. Taylor, and R. Wensel. 1994. *Organizational Transformation in Healthcare: A Work in Progress.* San Francisco: Jossey-Bass.

Appelbaum, S. H. 1997. "Socio-Technical Systems Theory: An Intervention Strategy for Organizational Development." *Management Decision* 35 (6): 452–63.

Center for the Study of Healthcare Management. 2002. *Designing a Safe Hospital.* Minneapolis, MN: CSHM.

Christensen, M. C., R. Bohmer, and J. Kenagy. 2000. "Will Disruptive Innovations Cure Health Care?" *Harvard Business Review* (September/October: 102–12.

Copeland, Y., L. B. Johnson, and R. Orr. 1997. "Opening the Gateway to Change: Creating a Human-Centered Medical Center—Strategies for Competing in the Healthcare Marketplace." *Journal of Healthcare Design* 9 (1): 105–08.

Hamilton, D. K. 2003. "Design of Patient Units and Organizational Performance." Master's thesis, Pepperdine University, Malibu, California.

Mallak, L. A., D. M. Lyth, S. D. Olson, S. M. Ulshafer, and F. Sardone. 2003a. "Culture, the Built Environment, and Healthcare Organizational Performance." *Managing Service Quality* 13 (1): 27–38.

―――. 2003b. "Diagnosing Culture in Healthcare Organizations Using Critical Incidents." *International Journal of Health Care Quality Assurance* 16 (4): 180–90.

Schein, E. H. 1992. *Organizational Culture and Leadership, 2nd Edition.* San Francisco: Jossey-Bass.

RECOMMENDED READING

Baier, S. 1985. *Bed Number Ten.* New York: Holt, Rinehart and Winston.

Bate, P. 1994. *Strategies for Cultural Change.* Woburn, MA: Butterworth Heinemann.

Buckingham, M., and C. Coffman. 1999. *First Break All The Rules.* New York: Simon & Schuster.

Chapman, E. 2003. *Radical Loving Care: Building the Healing Hospital in America.* Franklin, TN: Providence House Publishers.

Cherns, A. 1976. "The Principles of Sociotechnical Design." *Human Relations* 29: 783–92. 29.

Coile, R. C. 2003. *Futurescan 2003: A Forecast of Healthcare Trends 2003–2007.* Chicago: Health Administration Press.

Frampton, S., L. Gilpin, and P. Charmel. 2003. *Putting Patients First: Designing and Practicing Patient-Centered Care.* San Francisco: Jossey-Bass.

Gerteis, M., S. Edgman-Levitan, J. Daley, and T. Delbanco. 1993. *Through the Patient's Eyes: Understanding and Promoting Patient-Centered Care.* San Francisco: Jossey-Bass.

Hamilton, D. K. 2002a. "Evidence-Based Design of Healthcare Facilities Improves Outcomes." *European Hospital Decisions* (August):

―――. 2002b. "First Design the Organization, then Design the Building!" *Interiors & Sources* (January/February): 94–95.

―――. 2002c. *Organization Theory and Healthcare Architecture.* Houston, TX: Center for Innovation in Health Facilities.

―――. 2003a. "Before Breaking Ground, Take Stock." *Modern Healthcare* (October): 6, 19.

―――. 2003b. "Relating Facility Design to Organization Design." *Healthcare Design* (September): 26–31.

Institute of Medicine. 2001. *Crossing the Quality Chasm: A New Health System for the 21st Century.* Washington, DC: National Academies Press.

Kelly, K. (ed.). 1995. *Health Care Work Redesign. Series on Nursing Administration.* Thousand Oaks, CA: Sage Publications.

Kotter, J. P. 1978. *Organizational Dynamics: Diagnosis and Intervention.* Reading, MA: Addison-Wesley.

———. 1996. *Leading Change.* Boston: Harvard Business School Press.

Lee, N. 2005. "Guidelines for the Design and Implementation of a Holistic, Patient-Family Centered Culture." Unpublished paper, St. Joseph Health System, Orange, California.

Malkin, J. 2002. "The Business Case for Creating a Healing Environment." *Board Room Press Newsletter* (October), 5–6.

Orr, R. 1989. "Healthcare Environments for Healing." *Journal of Health Care Interior Design* 1 (10): 71–76.

———. 1992. "The Planetree Philosophy." *Journal of Health Care Design* 5 (1): 29–34.

Press, I. 2002. *Patient Satisfaction: Defining, Measuring, and Improving the Experience of Care.* Chicago: Health Administration Press.

Rosen, R. 1991. *The Healthy Company: Eight Strategies to Develop People, Productivity and Profits.* New York: Jeremy P. Tarcher/Perigee Books.

Sadler, B. 2001. "Healthcare Design as a Strategic Advantage in a Competitive Managed Care Environment." In *Design & Health—The Therapeutic Benefits of Design,* edited by A. Dilani, 85–93. Stockholm: Svensk Byggtjänst.

Secretain, L. 1997. *Reclaiming Higher Ground.* New York: McGraw-Hill.

Steele, F. I. 1973. *Physical Settings and Organization Development.* Reading, MA: Addison-Wesley.

Ulrich, R. S. 1997. "A Theory of Supportive Design for Healthcare Facilities." *Journal of Healthcare Design* 10 (1): 3–7.

CHAPTER 9

The Vision Starts at the Top

Sara O. Marberry

So what does it really take to build an extraordinary hospital building? The healthcare organizations that have done it in the United States have at least one thing in common: an extraordinary leader who embraces and champions the vision of creating a healing environment for patients, staff, and visitors.

Connie Harmsen, Blair Sadler, and Frank Sardone are three such leaders. Their experiences, while similar in many ways, are also very different. Each will share their thoughts and feelings in this chapter. But first, a little background is necessary.

THREE EXEMPLARY ORGANIZATIONS

Children's Hospital and Health Center

Blair Sadler has served as president and CEO of Children's Hospital and Health Center in San Diego, California, since July 1980. Before that he was vice president and director of the hospital and clinics at Scripps Clinic and Research Foundation in La Jolla. An attorney by training, he began his career as a medicolegal specialist for the National Institutes of Health in Washington, DC; was a member of the Yale

University faculty; and served as an assistant vice president at the Robert Wood Johnson Foundation in Princeton, New Jersey.

Sadler was at the helm of Children's when its new Rose Pavilion was designed in the early 1990s and opened in January 1993. The building is the focal point of a 28-acre hospital campus that originally opened its doors in 1954 with additions built throughout the 1960s, 1970s, and 1980s. Facing an increasing patient population and steadily increasing market share, Children's Hospital found itself turning away patients in the 1980s because it did not have enough beds or outpatient clinic space. The decision was made to build a new children's hospital—one that looked and felt playful, calming, and homelike, not like a traditional hospital.

As an early adopter of some of the principles we now call evidence-based design, the 190,000-square-foot, 115-bed Rose Pavilion features such positive distractions as interactive art for children, outdoor courtyards, and midnight "starfields" in nursing units. Provisions for family members, such as comfortable waiting areas and in-room sleep areas, are also incorporated. Room identification through color association gives children a sense of control and personalization. Control is provided through the choice of art, lighting, temperature, noise, and meals. The building's distinctive exterior architecture is reflective of the San Diego area, and its variety of roofs and forms present an intriguing image to the community. A clock tower serves as a characteristic symbol of San Diego and its people, colors, and shapes (Carter et al. 1993).

The patient, family, and staff response to the new facility was extraordinarily positive. Children's Hospital quickly became the gold standard in the industry for children's hospital design and has received many awards. In the past ten years it also added more artwork and two healing gardens and has begun planning a major five-story addition that includes sixteen operating rooms, a new neonatal intensive care unit, and additional acute care beds. Originally planned as a freestanding hospital to replace its aging convalescent hospital—the only one in California for children—Children's Hospital undertook a comprehensive study of the existing facility to ascertain the level of family and caregiver satisfaction. The opportunity to take data from an existing facility and measure them against a new facility was what launched The Center for Health Design's Pebble Project initiative in 2000.

Because of financial constraints, construction of the new facilities was delayed. During that time, the number of children in this population who could be cared for at home has significantly increased, and the number needing hospitalization has decreased by one-third. Consequently, Children's Hospital has decided not to build the original freestanding hospital, but to renovate a different part of the hospital for this patient population after another project is completed. For its Pebble Project, Children's Hospital still intends to undertake a comprehensive analysis of the impact of the new environment on families and caregivers.

Eight years after the Rose Pavilion opened, Sadler saw the hospital's market share increase by 13 percent, and it became the preferred provider by 3.5 to 1 over the nearest competitor (The Center for Health Design 2002). In four years specialty outpatient volume increased by 70 percent, and the emergency care center, which was built in 1999 to accommodate 25,000 visits a year, exceeded 55,000 visits.

Reduced pricing, reduced costs, improved customer service, excellent demonstrated clinical outcomes because of dedicated staff, and the uniqueness of the built environment are the five factors Sadler (2001) attributes to this success. The impact of the Rose Pavilion's innovative design was also instrumental in raising $5 million during and immediately following construction (Berry et al. 2004). Sadler (2001) insists that the "lesson for healthcare organizations is clear—provide a built environment that is welcoming to patients, improves their quality of life, and supports families and employees or suffer the economic consequences in a competitive environment."

Bronson Healthcare Group

An MBA-educated executive, Frank Sardone joined Bronson Healthcare Group in 1988. Over the next eight years he served in various roles, including chief operating officer, before becoming president and CEO in 1996. At that time he assumed leadership of the development of a $181 million project that began in 1993 to redevelop Bronson's 100-year-old Kalamazoo, Michigan, campus.

Since its founding in 1901, Bronson had expanded to tightly fill four city blocks with no green space or circulation through the campus. Early on, the board made the decision to maintain Bronson's commitment to downtown Kalamazoo. After studies showed that Bronson could save $50 million by building a new facility instead of renovating the existing facility, the management team decided to build on a 14-acre site across from the existing facility. The board and management team realized that they had a rare opportunity to "do it right" and started to rethink what they were doing.

This mind-set shift sent them down a new path with the goals of creating a healing environment, enhancing customer service, inspiring and transforming the culture, and improving performance. In April 2000 a new medical office pavilion and outpatient pavilion opened, followed by a new 750,000-square-foot inpatient hospital in December. A large indoor atrium garden is the centerpiece of the new hospital, providing that much-needed connection to nature and access to natural light. It features 20 varieties of plants and a total of 1,500 plantings. The open circulation of the building, along with limited internal corridors, a balance of natural and artificial light, and places for activity and rest, facilitates intuitive wayfinding. Earth tones and a natural color palette combine with organic patterns and natural materials to soften the clinical atmosphere of waiting areas and patient units. Private rooms have landscape views as well as space for the provider, patient, and family, plus a separate hand-washing sink for staff (Sardone et al. 2000).

Customer service has been enhanced by the proximity of the hospital to the medical pavilion as well as the convenient parking and the vertical and horizontal alignment of the buildings. A culture assessment study showed that the new building's design provides a layout and environment that allow caregivers to meet patient needs better than they could in the old facility. The value of a strong culture, one in which people know and accept the organization's values and in which their behavior consistently illustrates the values of the organization, was also revealed (Mallak et al. 2002).

As another early adopter of evidence-based design, Sardone has often commented that when Bronson began its project in 1993, there was little evidence that any of these design innovations would have positive outcomes. By joining the Pebble Project research initiative in 2001 after its project was complete, Bronson has been able to quickly contribute to the body of evidence in a meaningful way. For example, nursing turnover rates are just 6.5 percent, and overall patient satisfaction has increased to more than 95 percent. Nosocomial infection rates declined by about 10 percent in the two years after the move because of the private room design, and market share increased by more than 2 percent (Berry et al. 2004).

Bronson has garnered an impressive collection of awards and honors not only for the new facility but also for excellence in patient care and the quality of its workforce. Among them are receiving Arbor Associates Award for Highest Overall Patient Satisfaction for four consecutive years; being named to *Fortune* magazine's list of the "100 Best Companies to Work For" (2004, 2005) and *Working Mother's* "100 Best Companies for Working Mothers" (2003, 2004, 2005); and receiving the Michigan Quality Leadership Award, the state equivalent of the national Baldrige award, in 2001.

Banner Estrella Medical Center

Banner Estrella Medical Center CEO Connie Harmsen began her professional career in the Midwest as a nursing assistant, clinical nurse, nurse practitioner, and nurse educator. After getting a master's degree in hospital administration, she worked as an administrator in Illinois, New Mexico, and Arizona, including serving as chief operating officer for Banner Good Samaritan Medical Center in Phoenix. In 2002 she became the first employee and CEO of Banner Estrella Medical Center, when Banner Health decided to build a new hospital on a greenfield site on Phoenix's rapidly growing west side.

Unlike those of Children's Hospital or Bronson, Harmsen's building project was begun completely from scratch. In addition, it was to be a model for other new hospitals to be built by Banner Health, already the leading provider of healthcare in the Phoenix area. After breaking ground in February 2003, the new 172-bed hospital was completed just 22 months later, officially opening its doors in January

2005. It sits on a 50-acre site that has a connected five-story medical office building and a freestanding 16,000-square-foot outpatient surgery center.

Built as a "hospital for the future," Banner Estrella is designed and constructed to be flexible and adaptable so it can evolve with changes and advances in medicine. Major infrastructure is routed along the perimeter of the buildings to allow for relatively easy reconfiguration of interior walls and spaces as demand for certain types of services increases or decreases. In addition, a below-grade access corridor, or spine, runs along the entire length of the hospital's main building, allowing up to two additional patient towers to be built along the spine and literally plugged in as they are completed with little or no impact to the existing hospital. The campus is also configured in such a way that all future expansion will take place behind the hospital so entrances and existing patient rooms are not affected.

The hospital is also designed to incorporate state-of-the art electronic medical records (EMRs), a computerized physician order entry system (CPOE), and telemedicine capabilities. CPOE allows physicians to place medication orders and other instructions electronically, a method that increases patient safety. To further decrease medication errors the hospital has brightly lit, enclosed medication rooms to reduce interruptions and distractions and decentralized alcoves and nursing stations to enable physician and staff to document patient information near the point of care.

Reflecting the importance of the role that family and friends play in patients' health, Banner Estrella also has large patient-family suites on each of its patient care floors. Each suite is private, complete with a restroom; couch that folds into a twin bed; and 30-inch flat-screen television that provides access to local programming, cable television channels, educational videos, Internet access, games, and pay-per-view movies. Suites are designed using the universal room concept, allowing for most patients to remain in one room during their entire stay. Headboards hide medical equipment so that the rooms feel less like hospital rooms and more like bedrooms. Patients can also choose the art for their room.

To ensure that family members remain strong for their loved ones who need care, Banner Estrella offers them a variety of services, including massage therapy and acupuncture.

Also a member of the Pebble Project, Banner Estrella is just beginning to collect data on medication errors, patient falls, nosocomial infections, caregiver turnover, teamwork, staff satisfaction, and patient satisfaction. Because Banner Estrella is a new facility, Harmsen and her team plan to benchmark these data against those of other Banner Health hospitals. However, in the first three months of opening patient satisfaction was in the 99th percentile, and staff satisfaction was in the 88th percentile. The hospital has also been performing monthly staff surveys to assess culture issues as well as collecting stories about the staff's personal experiences, patient care experiences, the physical environment, and the technological environment. A teamwork survey done in January 2005 showed a high level of job enjoyment, clarity about goals and contributions to the mission, an emerging commitment to creating a world-class hospital, and growing team cohesion (Harmsen and Malloch 2005).

THE LEADERS SHARE THEIR EXPERIENCES

Harmsen, Sadler, and Sardone sat down together and talked about their experiences of building new hospital buildings. The rest of this chapter is a summary of their discussion.

What Made You Decide to Build an Extraordinary Hospital Building?

Sadler: The turning point for me was the day in 1991 when our architects, NBBJ, told a group of us during a meeting that they wanted to play a game with us. So the five of us—a board leader, two physician leaders, the vice president of planning, and me—sat around the table with the two lead architects, who handed out a series of 3 × 5-inch cards. They told us they were going to ask us a single question that they hadn't asked before, and that they wanted us to react quickly and write down what came to us on the cards. The question was, "What do you want this new hospital pavilion to *feel* like?" Well, we had never really thought about this, but we filled out the cards and put all of them up on the wall. They clustered into eight feelings:

childlike, playful, honest, homelike, friendly, nonintimidating, consistent with San Diego architecture and environment, and a place where people like to work. And they asked us, "Do you really believe this? Is this what you really want?" We did a quick gut check and decided that we did, and it drove the vision for creating something very special—something that felt very authentic to us because it was consistent with the values of the organization.

I probably didn't know it at the time, but talking about what we wanted the hospital to feel like was something much more personal for me. I'd heard healthcare futurist Leland Kaiser speak the previous year. He touches feelings, and his message resonated with me because, as a trained lawyer, part of what I love most about my job is being an advocate for kids, particularly poor kids. Why shouldn't every kid have a healthcare experience that is the same as every other kid? I'm also a cancer survivor and had spent some time at a major teaching hospital on the East Coast that was definitely not a healing environment. We had to fight with housekeeping just to put a poster on the wall. So thinking about what we wanted the hospital to feel like and connecting it to my own experiences drove the vision for creating something very special.

Harmsen: I knew from the start that I wanted to create a healing environment. About 15 years ago, I had attended a leadership conference in which we did some guided imagery and visioning exercises. During one of these exercises, I envisioned a healing environment that was unlike any I had seen or experienced before. It wasn't going to be easy creating it, and we as an organization would have to show a lot of courage to make it happen. There are a lot of risks that come with doing things differently.

The opportunity to create this new healing environment occurred shortly after we announced plans to build a new hospital in west Phoenix. It was to be a brand-new hospital on a greenfield site, so anything was possible. I was offered the job of CEO and instructed by the president of Banner Health to "create the hospital of the future." And we did. We began in early 2002 with a visioning conference that included board members, physicians, the best and brightest from across Banner Health, and healthcare futurists such as Charles Arntzen, Jeffrey Bauer, Kent Bottles, Leanne Kaiser Carlson,

Bill Dwyer, and Wanda Jones to help us explore the possibilities.

Together we decided that the hospital for the future had to be flexible and adaptable to meet our needs not only today, but in 20 years. It needed to have an EMR, CPOE, and telemedicine. We wanted to provide high-quality, safe care and have the highest service excellence for our patients and our associates. And it also had to be a healing environment.

Sardone: The biggest issue was that our facility was 100 years old. A couple of years before, we had set out on the path to renovate and we never even thought about the possibility of building a new facility. Our mind-set was renovation, which we had done about every 20 years or so. We had never thought about the possibility of whether we should start from scratch. We had done some studies that indicated that we could actually save about $50 million by building a new facility as opposed to renovating the old. This was a major epiphany for us. Once we made that big leap in thinking from remodeling an old facility to building a new, it became a once-in-a-lifetime opportunity to do it right. We started to rethink everything we were doing—from processes to how to develop a more patient-focused culture. It opened up everyone's minds about what the possibilities could be for totally reinventing the healthcare experience.

I was actually chief operating officer for Bronson when planning for the project started. Our CEO, Pat Ludwig, passed away before the project broke ground. He had an engineering background, and one of his major concerns was efficiency. Together we had done a fair amount of work with the board convincing them that building a new facility was the right thing to do, but always doing it against a backdrop of efficiency and making it clear that we felt we could actually reduce healthcare costs this way.

In the early 1990s very few organizations were building new hospitals. Many of our colleagues in the industry thought we were crazy. But, similar to Blair's experience, our creativity was charged after we started to work with our architects, Shepley Bulfinch Richardson and Abbott. We talked about convenience and creating a customer-oriented facility and what the hospital of the future should look like. In our case an extraordinary facility was the result of unleashing the creativity of a whole team of people committed to a new vision.

What Kind of Internal or External Resistance Did You Encounter?

Sadler: There was little expressed internal resistance to our project until the very end, when the board asked me several times, "Is this more expensive than it needs to be?" They wanted it to be in the median of other hospitals being built in the San Diego area. One board member even said at one point, "I want to be sure we can afford this gingerbread." What we were building was fundamentally different from the other hospitals in the area. In the end our project came in at the same square-foot cost of a nearby hospital opening a few months earlier.

 Harmsen: There was a lot of excitement about designing and building a new hospital, and everyone had their idea of what it should be. Gathering all the ideas, then making the best decisions about the specific details, was challenging. Moving into the facility, establishing the EMR and CPOE, orienting hundreds of staff, successfully passing the regulatory certifications, opening the hospital, and operating a safe, quality hospital was arduous work for many people. Banner Estrella was truly a cocreation by our entire Banner Health system.

 Sardone: The whole cost issue was also an incredible burden for us. The initial reaction from many in our community was, "How can you be spending these kind of dollars on a new facility when healthcare costs are already so high?" Also, from a timing standpoint, we had just completed a major workforce reduction and were concerned about the perception of trading "bodies for bricks." We spent a lot of time and effort educating the people in our community about how this was the right thing to do from both a cost and improvement in patient care standpoint.

Did You Ever Have Any Moments of Indecision?

Sadler: Five weeks before the Rose Pavilion opened, when everything was taking its final shape, I asked our vice president of facilities to try and gauge how people at Children's were feeling about the project. He came back to me and said, "I do not know how to tell you this, but it is not going well. This is so different from any hospital that anyone has ever seen that they think Sadler has gone crazy. In fact, somebody even called it 'Sadler's Folly.' They are saying that this does not feel like a hospital." And so even though we designed the hospital with everyone's input and let them know from the very beginning what we were doing, they felt this way. I became anxious and depressed to hear this and began wondering if we were doing the right thing, but a key colleague assured me that it would be okay.

And it was. In the four- to five-day time period after the building opened and before the kids moved in, the local media gave us extraordinary publicity. Crowds of people from the San Diego community came to see the new hospital. We ran out of brochures. One elderly couple told me after they took a tour, "We're so glad we got to see this. But there is just one thing that makes us sad. Why can't every other hospital in San Diego feel like this?" On that day and at that moment I felt vindicated. I'll never forget it.

Harmsen: I always thought that I was doing the right thing, but I didn't exactly know how to do it in the beginning. For the first year I was the only employee at Banner Estrella, and it was extremely lonely. My biggest challenge was holding onto the vision and believing that it was the right thing to do.

In August 2003, in my second year as Banner Estrella's CEO, I went to my first Pebble Project partner meeting. I knew I had met soulmates, and my vision was validated. After that we were able to engage the experienced engineering consultants at Starizon to help create our vision.

The other thing was that when there were moments of questioning, I sought advice from the right people. My experience as a clinician and a chief operating officer was invaluable in helping me to find those people. I also relied on my spiritual strength and trusted my intuitive feelings and honed in on that knowledge.

Sadler: Intuition was important for me, too. At one point when I felt scared and lonely, I called Leland Kaiser and shared my doubts. He told me to trust my feelings.

Sardone: There weren't many moments of indecision, just hurdles to cross. As I mentioned before, we anticipated push-back from the community on the project's $181 million cost. We too were worried about how the community was going to react to it. It was the largest building project the community had ever experienced. How were people going to react to us tearing down the old facility? We did a door-to-door campaign in the neighborhood to make sure people understood that this was something that was going to enhance rather than destroy their neighborhood.

Also, we had made it clear to people that we were not going to have any further workforce reductions when we moved into the new facility. We were a little nervous about whether we would be able to fulfill this promise. But prior to moving into the new facility we started customer service training with our employees and became much more customer focused. We actually saw an increase in our patients' satisfaction during this time. Our cultural transformation also began then, and we were able to engage the workforce and get them excited about the new facility. Also, we built the new parking garage first, so when employees got to work, they walked by the project every day and could visually see its progress. At one point we started doing tours for employees so by the time we opened the new building, everyone had been through multiple times and was comfortable with it.

What Was the Impact of Your New Hospital on Your Community?

Sadler: It was transforming. Children's became the talk of the community. Our employees were excited, our patients were happy, our families were empowered. We gained everyone's respect and admiration. We started winning awards and achieving recognition in the larger healthcare industry. This led me to The Center for Health Design, and it changed my whole journey. Also, the new building had an important impact on philanthropy. More people began to give to Children's, and even today, 12 years after the building was built, people who see the facility for the first time tell us, "You really are living your mission, aren't you?" Nurses and physicians have come to work at Children's because of the work environment, and our market share has increased significantly because of the culture of caring that is embodied by the building design. People write things on the open-ended questions on our customer satisfaction surveys like, "Our child cried when he went home. He thought it was Club Med."

Gina Wright, a writer who was doing a story on our healing gardens, spent considerable time walking around Children's. She concluded her article in *Décor & Style Magazine* by writing, "I know that I shall never get Children's Hospital out of my system. I have been back several times—it is a wonderful and inspiring place to visit even if one does not have a particular reason to be there" (Wright 2001). I guess this is about as good a statement of impact of our environment as I could ever wish for.

Harmsen: We've been open for three months, and our patient and employee satisfaction rates are high. We brought 800 new jobs to the West Valley, and our overall economic impact on the community is about $20 million a year. I hear many comments from people that the hospital isn't like any other that they've seen before. We have had no problem hiring nurses; they come to us because they resonate with the culture. Our hospital design is the prototype for all future Banner hospitals and has attracted attention from hospital providers across the country, many of whom have come to tour our facility and learn from us. Our patient care family room has also been extremely well-received by patients, families, our associates, and our physicians. It is a safer and more comfortable room that is a core element of the healing environment. The CPOE and EMR systems have also met our expectations well.

Sardone: By the time we broke ground on our project, there was a sense that it was a good thing—a catalyst to a downtown renaissance. Our project spurred streetscape improvements and small-business start-ups, enabled the city to build a new justice center on the site of our former outpatient surgery center, and was the beginning of a lot of new investment—both public and private—in downtown Kalamazoo. I think our project stabilized the downtown area and gave more people confidence to invest in keeping or starting businesses in this area. It definitely had a positive economic impact.

What Advice Would You Give Other CEOs Contemplating a New Building Project?

Sadler: The good news is that there is now lots of compelling, published evidence that doing it right—building a better building—improves the quality of healthcare, enhances safety, reduces errors, and improves workforce retention. Further, there is now evidence that operating cost savings offset and exceed the one-time capital costs for a better building, making it a superb long-term investment. So do your homework and learn all about the evidence. Also, recognize the connection between building a better building and being a responsible steward of scarce community resources. In other words, what you need to tell your community is, "We have thought about this carefully, reviewed the evidence, and it is a lot of money, but in the long-term it will save money and be a better use of our resources." The responsible CEO and board can't afford to not look at this evidence and do the right thing. Everybody wins.

Recognize that this may be the single most important opportunity you have in your career to leave a lasting legacy that helps your organization and your community. While it will be scary, lonely, and tiring to really push the envelope, if you get great advisors, paint a compelling future vision, and never give in, you will be participating in one of the most satisfying experiences in your professional life.

Harmsen: You need to have a vision, and it needs to be a grand vision of what you and your team, associates, physicians, and community can do working together. There are many ways to create a healing environment; the real issue is intention.

Sardone: Use building projects as a forum for change and to raise the bar. Step back and look at the big picture to make it something broader than the physical structure. And always look at the project from the patient and customer perspective. Consider the building to be a community asset, something that is an integral part of the community.

REFERENCES

Berry, L., D. Parker, R. Coile, D. K. Hamilton, D. O'Neill, and B. Sadler. 2004. "The Business Base for Better Buildings." *Frontiers of Health Services Management* 21 (1): 3–24.

Carter, E., D. Noferi, A. Ridernour, B. Sadler, and D. Swain. 1993. "San Diego Children's Hospital & Health Center Addition." *Journal of Healthcare Design* 5 (1): 25–31.

The Center for Health Design. 2002. "Competing by Design." Presented at an executive program sponsored by Turner Healthcare, Indianapolis, Indiana. October 11.

Harmsen, C., and K. Malloch. 2005. "Banner Estrella Medical Center Pebble Project Update." Presented at a Pebble Project partner meeting, Orlando, Florida, March 31.

Mallak, L., S. Olson, S. Ulshafer, and F. Sardone. 2002. "Bronson Has Designs on Culture Change." *Healthcare Design* (September): 26–29.

Sadler, B. 2001. "Design to Compete in Managed Care." *Facilities Design & Management* (March): 38–41.

Sardone, F., J. Dixon, E. Ericson, and J. Gyory. 2000. "The New Bronson Methodist Hospital." Presented at the Symposium on Healthcare Design, Anaheim, California, December 1.

Wright, G. 2001. "Hospital Gardens and their Effect on Patients." *Décor and Style* (July): 44–46, 54, 56.

About the Contributors

EDITOR

Sara O. Marberry is president of Sara Marberry Communications, a consulting firm in Evanston, Illinois, that provides writing, editing, and marketing services for the healthcare and design industry. She has worked as a consultant to the Symposium on Healthcare Design/The Center for Health Design since 1990 and is currently The Center's director of communications. Ms. Marberry is a former editor of *Contract* magazine and was also a communications coordinator for the world's largest design center, the Merchandise Mart in Chicago. She is the editor of Volumes III to X of the *Journal of Healthcare Design*, author of *Color in the Office: Design Trends from 1950–1990 and Beyond*, coauthor of *The Power of Color: Creating Healthy Interior Spaces*, editor of *Innovations in Healthcare: Selected Presentations from the First Five Symposia on Healthcare Design*, and editor of *Healthcare Design: An Introduction*.

CONTRIBUTING AUTHORS

Leonard L. Berry, Ph.D., is distinguished professor of marketing and holds the M. B. Zale Chair in Retailing and Marketing Leadership in the Mays Business School at Texas A&M University. He is also professor of Humanities in Medicine in the College of Medicine at Texas A&M University System Health Science Center. During the 2001–2002 academic term, he served as a visiting scientist at Mayo Clinic studying healthcare service. He is the founder of Texas A&M's Center for Retailing Studies and served as its director from 1982 to 2000. A member of The Center for Health Design's board of directors, he is a former national president of the American Marketing Association.

Rosalyn Cama, FASID, is president and principal interior designer of Cama, Inc., in New Haven, Connecticut. An interior planning and design firm steeped in evidence-base design, the firm's mission is to create interior environments that improve the human experience. Ms. Cama has been a practicing healthcare designer for Baystate Health System, Yale-New Haven Hospital, Riley Outpatient Center, and OhioHealth. A fellow of the American Society of Interior Designers (ASID), Ms. Cama is the chair of The Center for Health Design's board of directors, has served as the chair of the ASID Healthcare Specialty Network, and is a past ASID national president.

Paul Alexander Clark, M.P.A., is senior knowledge manager for Press Ganey Associates in South Bend, Indiana. Press Ganey partners with healthcare organizations to measure and improve the satisfaction of their customers, including patients, residents, physicians, and employees. Mr. Clark directs a team that proactively conducts qualitative and quantitative research to provide real-time knowledge support for hundreds of Press Ganey consultants. His research is published regularly in peer-reviewed journals.

Robin Guenther, AIA, LEED AP, ASHE, is the principal of Guenther 5 Architects, a New York City firm with extensive experience in healthcare design. Her projects have received national design awards and have been widely published. She is a member of the 2006 AIA Guidelines for Healthcare Construction Revision Committee, the steering committee of the Green Guide for Health Care, and the LEED for Healthcare Application Guide Core Committee. She is also a member of The Center for Health Design's Environmental Standards Council.

D. Kirk Hamilton, FAIA, FACHA, is a fellow of The Center for Health Systems & Design and associate professor of architecture at Texas A&M University in College Station, where his research area is the relationship between evidence-based design of health facilities and measurable organizational performance. He is also a founding principal of WHR Architects in Houston and Dallas and serves on The Center for Health Design's board of directors.

Connie Harmsen is the former CEO of Banner Estrella Medical Center in Phoenix. She began her professional career in the Midwest as a nursing assistant, clinical nurse, nurse practitioner, and nurse educator, with cardiac care as her specialty. After getting a master's degree in hospital administration from the University of Minnesota, Ms. Harmsen moved into hospital management, working as an administrator in Illinois, New Mexico, and Arizona. Prior to her appointment at Banner Estrella, she was the chief operating officer of Banner Good Samaritan Medical Center in Phoenix.

Anjali Joseph, M.A., is the director of research at The Center for Health Design in Concord, California. She is a Ph.D. candidate in architecture from the Georgia Institute of Technology, where she minored in health systems. She also holds a master's degree from Kansas State University. Dr. Joseph is responsible for coordinating the research activities of The Center's Pebble Project partners and supports their evidence-based design efforts.

Jain Malkin is president of Jain Malkin, Inc., a San Diego interior architecture firm specializing in healthcare facilities. A leader in the field of healthcare design, Ms. Malkin has lectured widely and written numerous articles on the psychological effects of healthcare environments. She teaches at Harvard University in the Graduate School of Design and is often a keynote speaker at conferences on the design of healing environments. Ms. Malkin is the author of several books on healthcare design, including *Medical and Dental Space Planning: A Comprehensive Guide to Design, Equipment, and Clinical Procedures* and *Hospital Interior Architecture*. She is a founding member of The Center for Health Design's board of directors.

Mary P. Malone, M.S., J.D., is president of Malone Advisory Services in South Bend, Indiana. She has more than 20 years of experience in the healthcare industry. Prior to forming her own firm, she worked for Press Ganey Associates, the nation's largest healthcare satisfaction measurement and improvement company, for more than 14 years, serving in a variety of senior leadership positions in corporate development, marketing, communications, customer service, and sales. She was responsible for integrating the operations of the former Parkside Associates, which was purchased by Press Ganey. Ms. Malone is a member of The Center for Health Design's board of directors.

Robin Diane Orr, M.P.H., is president of the Robin Orr Group, a Santa Barbara, California-based consulting firm that provides organizational consulting services to healthcare providers, architects, interior designers, and product manufacturers. She was a founding member of The Center for Health Design's board of directors and is the former executive director and national director of hospital projects for Planetree, an international organization known for its humanistic, patient-oriented approach to healthcare delivery and information access.

Derek Parker, FAIA, RIBA, FACHA, is director of Anshen + Allen Architects, with offices in San Francisco, Los Angeles, Seattle, Salt Lake City, and Baltimore, and chair of Anshen Dyer of London and Manchester. An internationally recognized expert in the design of healthcare and research facilities, Mr. Parker has designed and planned more than 50 major hospitals, diagnostic care centers, hospices, and medical research institutes in his 43 years with the firm. He is a founding member of The Center for Health Design's board of directors.

Xiaobo Quan, M.Arch, is a Ph.D. candidate at College of Architecture at Texas A&M University. He has a bachelor and master's degree in architecture from Southeast University at Nanjing, China. His master's thesis focused on the assisted housing and nursing homes for elderly people in Nanjing City. Together with other team members, he won the first prize of the "Year 2000 Urban & Rural Affordable Housing" international design competition in 1996. From 1997 to 2001 he worked with Shanghai Xian Dai Architectural Design (Group) Co. Ltd. In 2001 he began his study at Texas A&M University, focusing on healthcare design.

Greg L. Roberts, AIA, FCSI, CCS, CCCA, LEED AP, ACHA, is a principal and director of specifications with WHR Architects, a firm specializing in healthcare architecture in Houston and Dallas. He is past chair of the Texas Society of Architects' Sustainable Environment Committee and served on the Construction Specifications Institute's Environmental Task Team, a national team charged with developing guidelines for "greening" the institute. He also serves on the steering committee of the Green Guide for Health Care and the Core Committee of the LEED Application Guide for Healthcare Facilities, two national initiatives focused on green healthcare facilities. Mr. Roberts is a director for the Greater Houston Area chapter of the U.S. Green Buildings Council and chairs its Education Committee. He also serves as director of knowledge communities on the American Institute of Architects Houston board of directors.

Blair L. Sadler, J.D., has been president and CEO of San Diego's Children's Hospital and Health since 1980. A graduate of Amherst College and the University of Pennsylvania Law School, he served as a medical-legal specialist for the National Institutes for Health, on the Yale faculty, and as assistant vice president at the Robert Wood Johnson Foundation. Prior to his appointment at Children's Hospital, Mr. Sadler served as vice president and director of the hospital and clinics at Scripps Clinical and Research Foundation. He founded and chairs the Child Health Accountability Initiative (CHAI), a consortium of 15 children's hospitals dedicated to improving the health of America's children, and is on the National Quality Forum's steering committee on acute hospital measures. Mr. Sadler is also a member of The Center for Health Design's board of directors.

Frank J. Sardone is prsident and CEO of Bronson Healthcare Group, Inc., in Kalamazoo, Michigan. Established in 1900, Bronson has a long history of providing high-quality medical care to people throughout Southwest Michigan. With a workforce of 3,900, Bronson is Kalamazoo's second largest employer. Mr. Sardone received a bachelor of science degree in 1979 and a master's of business administration in 1981 from the University of Kentucky. He joined Bronson in 1988 and assumed his current role in 1996. Mr. Sardone is a member of The Center for Health Design's board of directors.

Roger S. Ulrich, Ph.D., is professor of architecture at Texas A&M University and a faculty fellow of The Center for Health Systems and Design, an interdisciplinary center housed jointly in the colleges of Architecture and Medicine. A behavioral scientist, he conducts research on the effects of healthcare facilities on safety and other medical outcomes. Among other achievements, his research is the first to scientifically document the health-related benefits patients experience by viewing nature. Dr. Ulrich has published widely in both scientific and design journals and is probably the most frequently cited researcher internationally in evidence-based healthcare design. His work has influenced the architecture, interior design, and site planning of scores of major hospitals in different countries. He is a founding member of The Center for Health Design's board of directors.

Craig Zimring, Ph.D., is an environmental psychologist and professor of architecture at the Georgia Institute of Technology in Atlanta. His work focuses on understanding the relationships between the physical environment and human satisfaction, health, performance, and behavior. Dr. Zimring has conducted studies for Steelcase, the Robert Wood Johnson Foundation, U.S. General Services Administration, Santa Clara County's Valley Medical Center, Ministry of Education of France, World Bank, California Department of Corrections, U.S. Courts, U.S. Department of State, Florida Board of Regents, California Department of General Services, Army Corps of Engineers, and many others. He is a member of The Center for Health Design's board of directors.

About The Center for Health Design

FOUNDED IN 1993, The Center for Health Design (The Center; www.healthdesign.org) is a not-for-profit research and advocacy organization based in Concord, California. Its mission is to transform healthcare settings into healing environments that improve outcomes through the creative use of evidence-based design. The Center's leaders and members envision a future in which healing environments are recognized as a vital part of therapeutic treatment and in which the design of healthcare settings contributes to health rather than adds to the burden of stress. The main areas of The Center's focus are research, education, environmental standards, and technical assistance.

The Center is committed to sharing the evidence-based knowledge gained through its Pebble Project field-study series in a timely fashion through programs such as the Turner Construction executive program series and partnerships with the Institute for Healthcare Improvement; the Robert Wood Johnson Foundation; Huda B. and Maurice L. Rothschild Foundation; and Medquest Communications, which, in association with The Center, publishes *Healthcare Design* magazine and produces an annual conference by the same name.

It is with great respect that The Center acknowledges its Pebble partners for their leadership and generosity to share their project results in a valid format.